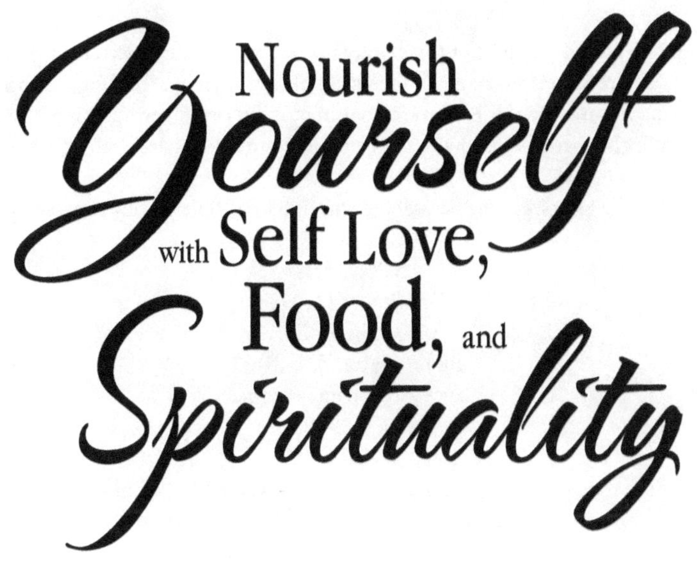

DEBORA ACCOLA

BALBOA.PRESS
A DIVISION OF HAY HOUSE

Balboa Press books may be ordered through booksellers or by contacting:

Balboa Press
A Division of Hay House
1663 Liberty Drive
Bloomington, IN 47403
www.balboapress.com
844-682-1282

Because of the dynamic nature of the Internet, any web addresses or links contained in this book may have changed since publication and may no longer be valid. The views expressed in this work are solely those of the author and do not necessarily reflect the views of the publisher, and the publisher hereby disclaims any responsibility for them.

The author of this book does not dispense medical advice or prescribe the use of any technique as a form of treatment for physical, emotional, or medical problems without the advice of a physician, either directly or indirectly. The intent of the author is only to offer information of a general nature to help you in your quest for emotional and spiritual well-being. In the event you use any of the information in this book for yourself, which is your constitutional right, the author and the publisher assume no responsibility for your actions.

Any people depicted in stock imagery provided by Getty Images are models, and such images are being used for illustrative purposes only. Certain stock imagery © Getty Images.

Print information available on the last page.

ISBN: 979-8-7652-2858-6 (sc)
ISBN: 979-8-7652-2859-3 (hc)
ISBN: 979-8-7652-2860-9 (e)

Library of Congress Control Number: 2022908447

Balboa Press rev. date: 05/09/2022

Contents

To my amazing kids, Mia and Noe:

Not only did you wake me up and show me that I
could live a life far better than I ever expected, but
you also made my life much more meaningful.

You fill every moment in my life with so much warmth and love.

You are my greatest teacher. I love you
both to the moon and back.

Thank you for choosing me as your mother; it means
the world to me. Thank you for giving me so much love
and thank you for being exactly the way you are.

Introduction

For years it has been one of my biggest dreams to write a book.

Now the time has come. I am sitting here at the computer writing my first book. I hope from the bottom of my heart that I will make a contribution to your life with *Nourish Yourself.* I truly believe that people pick up and read a specific book for a particular reason. I truly believe that higher power and our own power guides always steer us in the right direction when we have strayed from our path.

Often, I have experienced the situation of having bought a book and then not reading it at all or starting to read it many weeks or even months later because the time was simply not right before. That is why I believe we read books when we most need to hear what they have to say. We are guided to these books. It is as if a higher power speaks to us through a book.

Some books I have read several times. Whenever I need support, I intuitively reach for a particular book I've read in the past. This is another reason I am convinced that we are always guided. You might be holding *Nourish Yourself* in your hands right now for a reason. Whatever that reason is, I hope you will find the right message or answer within these pages and that you will be able to take from it what you need.

I am writing *Nourish Yourself* with the intention that it will become your daily source of spiritual food, along with being your guide to self-love and self-care.

How often do we get lost in the daily grind? How often do we get lost in the stories that we create in our heads? How often does it happen that we have time for everything but ourselves? How often do we wish for a hug, for someone to tell us everything is okay or will be okay? How often would we like a shoulder to lean on or just someone to talk to?

In *Nourish Yourself,* not only do you learn to be with yourself, connect with your body, and be present, but also, with the tools that I pass on to you, you learn to love yourself more, listen more to yourself and your body, let go of what blocks you, let the energy flow, and automatically come into your power.

I have noticed in myself, and I see it again and again with others, that without self-love and taking time for myself, no matter how healthily I eat or how much I exercise, I am missing a part of myself. The human body needs to move and needs food in order to function and remain alive, but it also needs self-love and self-care. It needs spiritual food because we are spiritual beings living in a physical body. The four aspects of a human being—body, mind, emotions, and spirit—are very closely connected to one another. If one part is out of balance, then the circle is incomplete. Often, I see that when a person works on self-love, then better nutrition automatically follows. When we love ourselves, it means we are more in our body, more connected to it. We pay more attention to ourselves, so we also sense what is really good for us and how much. We overeat less, we reach less often for processed foods, and our energy flows differently. Finally, it can flow through our bodies because we are no longer blocking ourselves.

With *Nourish Yourself,* my hope is that you will be more in your body, be connected to it, be in your power, and be inspired to follow your intuition. I hope that what you find within these pages will help you to strengthen your intuition, cause you to be less distracted by outside factors, and enable you to trust yourself and listen to your gut feeling. Basically, *Nourish Yourself* is about finding your power, learning to listen to yourself, and learning to trust yourself and your gut, or intuition. The tools herein are easy to implement in your daily life and incorporate step by step.

Always remember, you are exactly where you are supposed to be. Don't look to the right or to the left; go at your own pace, which may be slower or even faster than someone else's. Trust your journey; trust the chapter you are writing. We are all here for a special reason. We all have light within us that wants to shine. So, start today, here and now. Turn on your light and shine.

With *Nourish Yourself,* you will find your own way and gain the ability to navigate from the outside to the inside. No longer will you compare yourself to others or be distracted by external influences. You will begin to find your power and recognize how wonderful and unique you are.

My intention with *Nourish Yourself* is that I show you how to create and hold space for yourself. See *Nourish Yourself* as your guide, your support, your friend, your motivation, and your nourishment. Whatever you are looking for, whatever reason brought you to *Nourish Yourself,* it is important that you take from it what you need. *Nourish Yourself* is about you finding yourself, finding your power, and learning to listen to yourself and your body. It's about building a relationship with your body, giving it what it needs, so it can give you what you need and become the best version of yourself.

In *Nourish Yourself,* I share my own experiences and my knowledge as an integrative nutrition health coach and yoga instructor. I am not a doctor or a specialist. Everything I suggest to you within these pages, I do myself based on my own experience and my own knowledge as a health coach and Yoga Teacher. All the exercises and tools I share herein, I do myself. I share what helped me to become more grounded and to be in my own power. I share how I learned to listen to my intuition and trust it. The practical part of *Nourish Yourself* is easy to implement, and no prior knowledge is needed. The exercises within these pages can be done almost anywhere with little time or effort and can be integrated into your daily life. They all have the same goal: to bring you into your body and help you be in the here and now. They help you to be present so that you may come to love yourself and do good things for yourself.

I dedicated *Nourish Yourself* to my twins. The birth of my children woke me up. One could say that my own journey started with the birth of my twins. Back in my twenties, I struggled with severe digestive problems and hormonal issues. It wasn't until I decided to become a mother that the ball started rolling. The decision to become a mother unconsciously awakened something in me. This decision changed my life, first unconsciously, then very consciously. I sit here today proud to say that I am the person I always wanted to be, although I never believed I actually would achieve this. This is what I wish with all my heart for you as well. You have the right to be the person you want to be, and I hope that with the help of *Nourish Yourself,* you will find who that person is.

1

Food, Spirituality, and Self-Love: My Own Journey

When I changed my diet a few years ago because of my poor digestion, I quickly felt a positive change. Not only did I have better digestion, but also, I had more energy. My skin and hair texture improved as well.

In addition, I noticed how my self-care routine changed. The trigger was clearly the change in diet. With that, the ball automatically started rolling. With the change in diet, I made a commitment to myself, an invisible contract. I was ready to take better care of myself and do something good for myself. I didn't realize at the time that the change in my diet was just the trigger for much more to come. Nevertheless, it didn't take long before I noticed that I was paying more attention to myself. My self-care routine suddenly became more important. With this, my self-love and energy changed as well. I took more time for myself, no longer putting myself and my needs on the back burner. My whole being changed by my focusing on my body and its needs.

In chapter 3, I write more about food and energy. Food is energy for the human body. When I started changing my diet, my energy automatically changed. Instead of processed food, I chose fresh and unprocessed food, and this has energetically transferred to my whole being—one of the reasons why the changes I made didn't stop with my diet. Nutrition, self-love, and spirituality are intimately connected.

Maybe your journey started with self-love, and you also started paying more attention to what foods you chose and what you nourished your body with. How a journey start doesn't matter. The journey of self-love, the journey of eating the right food for your body, and the journey of spirituality all lead to the same place. Each of these journeys leads to you. They lead to your inner self.

Since I am convinced that one does not work without the others and that nutrition, spirituality, and self-love are firmly connected, *Nourish Yourself* is dedicated to these three areas. My goal with *Nourish Yourself* is that you may discover all three areas for yourself and find your balance. I hope that with what you read within these pages, you will find the way to yourself, get to know yourself, find your power, listen to yourself and your body—and trust it—and walk through your life in love.

My wish is that you find your uniqueness and come to know that you are allowed to put aside the idea of having to be perfect and show yourself as you are. No one is perfect. It took me a long time to realize this. I tend to be very hard on myself. As for me, I am a recovering perfectionist.

Today I live by the following mantra: "I am perfectly imperfect."

Of course, I still have moments when I fall into my old patterns. The exercises in *Nourish Yourself*—that I share with you here and also practice myself—allow me to recognize when I have fallen back into an old pattern and make a new choice. Doing these exercises help me change my perspective. They help me come into the present and be in my body.

My own journey started with making a resolution to improve my digestive problems and hormonal issues. After a few visits to the doctor, which unfortunately did not help me the way I had hoped, I resolved to change my diet. I was looking for changes that I could realistically implement. I didn't want to diet, I didn't want to forbid myself anything, yet I wanted to feel better. I began to eliminate processed foods step by step, as well as white flour and refined sugar. Even today I live according to the motto "Everything in balance." I am firmly convinced that what we do most of the time is more important than what we do now and then. I keep things that way today when it comes to food. I don't forbid myself anything, and sometimes I allow myself a cake that contains refined sugar or is baked with white flour. This is my way of being perfectly imperfect.

The change in diet helped me to learn to listen to my body. I was allowed to realize more and more that I resided too much in my masculine energy. I was ready to find the balance. In addition, I started to dedicate more time to my self-care routine. This, in turn, led to my journey toward spirituality. I started meditating, and the more I listened to my body, the more present I became, noticing my thoughts and emotions.

I saw in myself how nutrition, self-love, and spirituality were closely related, and I began to see the effects in my environment and even in my work.

Your journey may not start with nutrition as mine did. We are all on our own path. We are all going our own way, at our own pace, and we are all exactly where we need to be. Your journey may start with more mindfulness in everyday life, or it may start with more self-care. We all want, in the end, to achieve the right balance. We all want to feel good and step through the day full of energy.

This balance we strive for will be achieved with more mindfulness in our daily lives. By starting to listen to the signs our bodies give us, by listening to our bodies and giving them what they need, we help our bodies give us energy. We support them in their work, which makes us feel good. We support our whole being.

Are you ready to feel good? Are you ready to find the right balance for yourself? Do you want to be more mindful and have more self-love? If so, then I look forward to our journey together. I hope that *Nourish Yourself* will help you put the steps herein into action to improve yourself for the long run.

2

Self-Love

For a long time, I paid little attention to my own self-love. That is, I exercised regularly and practiced decent nutrition, but I was never truly satisfied with myself. I also never really realized how I was blocking myself and my body by my negative thoughts about my body and the poor way in which I spoke to myself. Our bodies not only process what we eat but also process and digest every word, every thought, and everything we experience. How we think about ourselves and what we say to ourselves are both hugely important when it comes to how we want to be, how we want to look, and how we want to perform.

I also failed to realize that how we relate to ourselves mirrors how we relate to other areas of our lives, for example, our relationship with food. In other words, our relationship with food can also be equated to how we think about ourselves.

Healthy eating and exercise are very important parts of our health and well-being. However, without the right mindset and the proper love and time for ourselves, we will always find something missing. We can't find love for ourselves anywhere but inside ourselves. That is why it is called *self-love.* No one can give you that. If you don't feel that love and you don't value yourself, no matter how slim, athletic, or good-looking you are, then you will always find that something is missing. That's why loving yourself and taking time for yourself is so important. They are necessary if you want to fill the circle so that no piece of the pie is missing. You can find happiness, love, and perfection only within yourself. You don't need anyone else for that. All you need is *yourself.*

Self-love and your relationship with food are closely related. It is also the case that your everyday life is influenced entirely by how well you love yourself.

Maybe you know this—those days when you are really dissatisfied with yourself, and you feel this dissatisfaction throughout your whole body. This automatically transfers to your mood, which transfers to your whole performance. You may just not be in a good mood. But you may also be transferring that mood to others, or that mood may be transferred to your work.

This is just one reason why it is important to love yourself. As I mentioned earlier, no one else can give you that love.

In this chapter, I go deeper into the topic of self-love. So often, to little attention is paid to this subject. You may be aware that self-love plays an important role and that you need to pay attention to cultivating it, but far too often your attention is given to something else, and self-love is put on the back burner.

To love yourself, you must nourish yourself daily. This means that you take time for yourself every day and do something good for yourself. This something good is different for everyone.

Maybe you already know what you need to do to love yourself more and take time for yourself. Maybe you lack practice, ideas, or time. The important thing is that you stay with yourself and don't become distracted by external influences. Today, the topics of wellness, self-care, and self-love are more present than ever. We all know how important they are. It is very easy to get lost when it comes to finding what is right for yourself. I remember a few months ago when the big supermarket in our area was remodeled. When I went shopping for the first time after the remodel, not only did I have to look all over for all the groceries I wanted but also, I was completely overwhelmed by the new offerings. Instead of a few plant-based milk alternatives, there were suddenly entire racks with countless plant-based milk alternatives. It was the same with the refined sugar-free granola bars. Where previously there were only two or maybe three varieties, there were suddenly entire racks full of granola and granola bars. It was completely overwhelming. I started studying the ingredients lists, but this got me nowhere because, first of all, most of the granolas had not only the same price but also almost the same ingredient list. They differed only very slightly. Second, I didn't have the time to study everything in detail. I listened to my gut feeling and reached for the product that intuitively appealed to me.

It is the same with wellness products on the market, such as granola or muesli bars. There are countless products, and many of them are similar and cost about the same. It is very difficult to find the right one. The same is true for something simple like a journal or a scented candle.

I want to stress to you that it doesn't take much to give yourself daily attention and nourish yourself and your body. One of my favorite mantras is "Back to basics." This goes for cooking and eating and also for self-care. "Less is more" could also be said here. It's not about your food having to be fancy, or your needing superfoods on your plate or a fancy sauce. It's the same with your self-care routine. You don't always need exclusive and expensive products. All you need is you and the love you have for yourself.

We dive deeper into self-love and self-care in this chapter. I will give you tools and action steps to integrate into your daily life, always with the focus that you do not lose yourself in too many external factors, but stay in your power, connect with your body, and be present.

Strengthen your love for yourself. Pay attention to your body. Nourish it from the inside and on the outside. If you do, you will see your intuition grow, along with your feminine power and your self-esteem.

2.1 **Where to start.**

What helped me personally when I decided to begin taking better care of myself and I didn't quite know where to start was to make a list of things I like to do. I wrote down both the small and large things that bring me joy and give me positive energy. While I was writing, I often closed my eyes and imagined things that really nourish me, things that give my body warmth and love. Then I wrote those things on my list.

Following are a few examples from my list:
- Reading a book.
- Drinking a hot chocolate.
- Getting a full-body massage.
- Playing with my children.
- Watching a romantic movie.
- Going out to eat at a restaurant of my choice and order without looking at the prices.

- Taking a spa weekend.
- Engaging in mindful movement.
- Taking a walk in nature.

I had deliberately chosen both expensive things and free things. Surprisingly, when I looked at the list, I discovered that most of the things on it were things that could be incorporated into my everyday life without any problem. Most of the things on the list were free or very inexpensive, such as drinking hot chocolate or playing with my kids. This showed me that it doesn't really take much to do something that gives me joy and nourishes my body and that I love doing.

You too can start a list. You may want to write it in your journal or on a piece of paper that you hang up in a place where you will see it often. Write a list of things that bring you joy. What have you always wanted to do? What fills your heart? What nourishes you on the inside?

For some, it may be watching a good romantic movie, as it is for me. For others, it is taking a bath. Still, others prefer simply lying on the sofa. The important thing here is that you write only what is right for you, not anyone else. Listen to your heart and intuition, and don't be influenced by external things.

As I mentioned before, my list surprisingly included many things that I had already integrated into my everyday life or that could be integrated easily. The only thing I needed to do was to prioritize these things and make time for them.

In this section, I help you find time for your self-care. You'll learn how to fit your self-care routine into your daily routine for the long term. You'll gain tips and tools for prioritizing yourself, and you'll learn to love yourself as a result.

Once you've made your list, go through your daily routine and think about where you can set aside some time each day and incorporate some of these new things.

If you're having a hard time finding time for yourself, think about your daily routine and ask yourself if you really need to watch TV as much every day or spend so much time on social media. Also, are there things you can put off until another day so you can carve out a window of time for these new things? Often people spend time on things they are not even aware of, such as watching TV for two hours in the evening. How about cutting that down to one and a half hours and setting aside half an hour for your self-care routine? Or you can schedule a time slot somewhere else.

Be worth it to yourself. You are the most important person in your life. You spend your whole life in your body, so respect it too. Treat it well and nurture it daily with lots of love and time for yourself. It's a matter of priorities. And believe me, I've had my priorities wrong many times. Look at how you can set your priorities. Taking time for yourself is not selfish. On the contrary, it brings you more into balance, makes you more satisfied, and causes you to feel more nourished—and your whole environment benefits from it.

Tips for Practicing Self-Love and Self-Care

Self-love plays an important role in every area of our lives, be it our relationship with food, our work, our home with family, or even our friendships.

Self-love is the foundation and the key to everything. If you don't love yourself, how can anyone else love you?

I have learned over the years that self-love is synonymous with accepting ourselves. We all have our good and bad points. No one is perfect, so we should stop trying to be perfect. It's exhausting and takes too much of our energy.

I invite you to accept yourself as you really are. Start today with a small task to nourish yourself and strengthen your self-love. Write down who you really are. Who is this person? Write down your desires and everything that comes through you. Take your time to do this. It's important not to get distracted and to go within to see what comes through.

I have a few tips for doing this exercise. First, find a quiet place. Maybe you like to light a candle to get yourself more in the mood to write. Breathe deeply in and out a few times. With each exhalation, visualize yourself going more and more into yourself, releasing all tension, and focusing only on your inner self. Feel free to close your eyes as you do this exercise. Then take a piece of paper or a journal and a pen and let the words come. Let it flow. Try to get out of your head and into your intuition. What would you like to put on the paper now? What are your deep desires? What does your I need? What does it want? How can you nourish it? How can you love it? Just write down what comes. Take all the time you need.

With this exercise, you gain access to your "me." Maybe things or desires come up that you never expected. Freewriting helps you to go deeper and discover what lies deep within you, what is hidden in your unconscious, and what you suppress or don't allow to come out in everyday life.

Put your paper in an envelope and keep it in a place of your choice. Or if you have written in your journal, keep it wherever you like.

Whenever you feel the need, go back and read the words you wrote down.

2.2 **How to find time for your self-care routine.**

If it is important enough for you, you will find a way.

We all have the same twenty-four hours each day. We can decide how we want to spend them.

I hear the same excuse over and over: "I'm busy" or "I don't have time to care for myself."

If something is important enough, we find the time for it. It's all a question of how and where we set our priorities.

Today I ask you to create space and time in your day for self-care. If you believe, or if you tell yourself, "I don't have time; my day is packed," then I ask you to write down everything you do, from the time you wake up to the time you go to bed. Write down when you take a shower or how long you spend on social media or watching Netflix. Write down how long your cooking takes or how long you spend attending to your household. Write down every task, and when you've finished, look at your list. What is on the list that can be eliminated or done on some other day? Where could you spend less time on something?

I ask you to go through your list and make room so that you have an hour leftover that you can use just for yourself.

Take your time when writing your list. It is very important that you not get overwhelmed. Take small steps. If you can't find one or two hours a day, then maybe you can find thirty minutes that you can dedicate to self-care.

If there is one thing I have learned over the past years, it is that as soon as I feel overwhelmed, I should take a step back and become the observer of the situation. Then I ask, "Why does this situation overwhelm me?"

Ask yourself the same question. Write the answer in your journal if you need to, and let the emotions come to the surface.

Sometimes when it comes to new routines, it can be very overwhelming. Please do not blame yourself if you feel overwhelmed by changing your routine or incorporating time for self-care.

Ask yourself, "How much do I want to feel good? How much do I want to take care of myself?"

The key is simply to start. If you can find only twenty minutes a day as a start, that's perfect. Once you create your new self-care routine, you will see that you create more time after a while. But if not, this is perfect too. There is no right or wrong. It is important that you find a way that works for you, not for anyone else.

2.3 What makes you truly happy?

Have you ever asked yourself this question? What is it that really brings you joy?

Take a moment, pick up your journal, and write down the things that bring you joy. Let the words flow. Feel the emotions that arise while you are writing the words. Maybe you will realize that something brings you much more joy than you realized before, or maybe something you thought brought you joy actually does not. Write down the little things too, such as walking barefoot or having a cup of tea or coffee. Whatever it is, try not to think about only the big things. Especially important are all the little things that bring joy to your life.

Wellness has become a big trend these days. We often see and read about what might be good for us. The truth is that only you know what is good for you.

After you write down your list of things that bring you joy, consider what you've written. Ask yourself how you can bring more joy into your life.

If you're struggling with this exercise and you don't know exactly what to write down, the following are a few tips to make writing easier:

Ensure that you are under no time pressure and that you are undisturbed. Close your eyes. Now imagine something that brings you a lot of joy. This can be going to a place such as a beach or your favorite coffee shop. Don't let yourself be restricted here; whatever comes up, let it emerge. Now immerse yourself in the feeling. What do you feel when you think of your favorite activity, favorite place, or something else that brings you joy? How does it feel in your body? Where do you feel something? Maybe you have a warm feeling in your body, or perhaps you have some butterflies in your stomach. Notice this feeling; allow it to happen; feel it deeply.

After a few minutes, slowly open your eyes. Sit for a while and feel your feelings.

Ask yourself the following question: "How do I feel when I am completely nourished from the inside out?"

Is it possible that this feeling is similar to the one you felt when you imagined the place that brings you joy?

Why do we love a place so much? Why do we love doing certain things, such as sitting and chatting with a girlfriend at our favorite coffee shop, or simply taking a bath? Because of the feeling that comes with it, that nurturing feeling that spreads throughout our bodies. This feeling makes us feel good, nourishes our bodies from the inside out, and gives our bodies love and energy.

Whenever you feel that you don't have enough time for yourself, whenever you are stressed, bored, or sad or you just need some me-time and self-care, remind yourself of the feeling. Whenever you feel that you need some self-love, take a few minutes and devote yourself to the following exercise:

Whenever necessary, ask yourself the question "How do I feel when I do the things I love or when I am in a place I love?"

While doing this, close your eyes and feel deep inside you. How does it feel when you are doing something you really love? Whenever you feel stressed or anxious, close your eyes and imagine yourself doing what you love or being in the place you love. Connect with that feeling. As you do so, take a few breaths in and out and really draw that feeling into your body, nourishing every cell.

We don't necessarily have to go to the beach. We don't necessarily have to leave where we are currently or book a spa appointment. Mostly we have to conjure up the feeling that is missing, the feeling we desire. Self-care is time for yourself, taking care of yourself. Self-care and self-love are connected. They belong together. You can always give yourself love by paying attention to yourself. Pay attention to how you feel. Where do you need self-care? What is missing from your life? When you give yourself a moment to do this exercise and connect with this nurturing feeling, you are giving pure love to your body and nourishment to your soul. You are taking care of yourself and doing something good for yourself, and you are doing it without having to go to the beach or visit an expensive spa. Everything you need is inside you. The answer, as so often, lies within you. Gift yourself love. Take a little time out whenever you need it, whether in the office, at home, or on the road. The exercise costs nothing. All it takes is you and your undivided attention to yourself.

2.4 **Self-care—how to build your healthy routine.**

In the previous section, you learned that everything you think you need is inside you.

Now we will talk about how a daily self-care routine is a foundation for your own balance. Humans are creatures of habit. We need security, and our daily routine gives us this security. What we do every day not only shapes who we are or who we become, ut also gives us the support, the ground, for our everyday life.

I remember when both my kids were babies, and their sleeping patterns changed every few months. It took me a few days each time to get into the new daily rhythm. Also, when the kids started kindergarten, our daily routine was completely restructured, and we all had to get used to it.

Maybe you know this already. When you are traveling, you are suddenly in a different time zone, or maybe you have a new job or children who start school. This change automatically brings with it a new daily routine, and you need time to get used to it. Routines are important because they provide support, balance, and grounding. They help you to reduce stress and become more centered.

But even though routines can be very supportive, sometimes daily routines have rather negative consequences on the body in the long run.

What is your goal? Who do you want to be? What can you implement daily to be that person? What does the person you've always wanted to be done every day? What are that person's aspirations? What does his or her daily routine look like?

Are your daily routines supportive of your long-term personal goals? Do they nourish your body? Do they sustain you and ground you in stressful times?

Feel free to take a few moments to reflect on these questions. You might also like to write the answers in your journal.

It's about what you do every day, what routines you have, and what you implement every day to be the person you want to be. The little things you do every day will ultimately get you to your goal. Therefore, connect your thoughts with the person you want to be. Take this energy into yourself.

Finally, ask yourself what you can do every day to reach your goal. What steps can you take, no matter how small they may be? Change leads to change. What can you change today to reach your goal?

To make it easier for you, I have a few tips for making long-term adjustments to your daily routines so that they support you in becoming the person you've always wanted to be.

Plant the seeds today in your daily routines today, and from now on you will be pouring water on your planted seeds, allowing them to grow and flourish. Remember, everything takes time. The journey is the destination. Whether your goal is to lose weight, live healthier, start your own business, or get pregnant, know that these things take time. Enjoy the moment, enjoy your path, and trust that it will lead you to your destination.

Following are some guidelines for implementing your new daily routine:

1. Make a Commitment to Yourself

How badly do you want to change your old habits?

How ready are you to create something new in your life?

Even if you get all the information, you need here, only you can make it happen—and only by making a commitment to yourself and wanting to achieve your goal. How much do you want to be the best version of yourself and feel good inside and out?

You can't create a successful company overnight. It takes daily work, and with every right step you take, you get a little closer to your goal. It's the same with your health or the body you want to have. You can't expect everything to have changed after a few weeks. It is the work you do every day to be the person you want to be that makes the difference. The important thing is that you show up for yourself every day. This means that even if there are days when you don't want to get up early to exercise, meditate, or make yourself a smoothie, you do it anyway—then you feel better afterward.

I too have days where I just want to eat chocolate, do nothing, and eat unhealthy food. But it's about what you do most of the time, not what you do once in a while. I always ask myself on those days, "How badly do I want to feel good? What is my why?"

I ask you to write down your why. Maybe hang it up somewhere on a wall or on the fridge as a daily reminder. That way you will have daily motivation to help yourself reach your goal.

Allow yourself to have bad days. Embrace each moment. Accept each moment as it is. The important thing is that you keep going. When you have a bad day, don't immediately think that all the work has been for nothing.

You will see that when you start doing good things for yourself on a daily basis, taking care of yourself, and incorporating routines such as daily exercise, daily meditation, or nourishing meals into your life, then not only does the change come, but also it becomes part of your being. Then it will always be easier to implement it because it belongs to you, and you embody it.

2. Balance Is the Key

As mentioned in point 1, we all have good days and bad days. What matters is what you we most of the time, not what we do once in a while.

I've noticed that the stricter I've been with myself in the past, the harder it has been for me to follow through.

If you forbid yourself and your body something, whether it is food (for example, chocolate or cake) or a break, then your body automatically demands more of the same. Children usually show us how this works. It is not for nothing that children are often the best teachers. If we don't allow them to do something, they want to do it even more. Think about finding balance. Enjoy your life. Enjoy every moment and embrace the good and the bad moments.

3. Go at Your Own Pace

Learning to go at my own pace was honestly not easy for me. I was constantly comparing myself to others, whether with regard to my work, my looks, or other things in my life. I was constantly comparing myself to others. With the advent of social media, it has become very difficult not to get lost and distracted by the outside world. However, it is more important than ever to stay with yourself. We all write our own books. We all go our own way. Your path is not comparable to the path of another person. Everyone has their own pace. Trust your path, write your chapter in the way that is right for you, and don't compare yourself to another person's book or chapter.

2.5 The power of breath.

Your Breath Should Be Your Best Friend

The more you connect with your breath, the more your body is able to relax. The more your body can relax, the more you can be. By connecting with your breath, you are not only supporting your nervous system but also allowing yourself to receive.

You can't receive the positive things of life if you try to bring them into your life from a place of stress.

When your body is in survival mode, that is, in stress mode and moving, there is no room for your body to be, and then there is no room for you to receive what you want to bring into your life.

When you are in a state of tension or stress, your body's energy is also stressed and tense, and there is compulsion behind your actions. Maybe you know that what you radiate energetically, you also attract.

You may be able to achieve certain goals in a stressful state. You may attract certain things into your life, and you may succeed. But the energy behind it is always the same, which is an energy based on stress. You bring these things into your life, for example, success, by way of stressed and tense energy. This causes you to invite more of that energy into your life. What if you could invite the things you want into your life with relaxed energy? How would your whole being change? How would it be if you were able to switch from stress mode to relax mode more often?

The nervous system, like everything else, needs balance. However, if you are always acting stressed and being in stress mode, then not only is your breath fast and shallow, but also your immune system is negatively affected, along with your thoughts, your whole system, your well-being, and your health.

It is very important that you recover and give yourself rest, not only for your nervous system, but also for your whole body system, your well-being, and your health.

Following are a few action steps and exercises that you can easily integrate into your everyday life. They will help you to bring your nervous system into relax mode, causing you to better inhabit your body. The more you are in your body, the calmer you are, the more you have access to your power and your intuition, and the more present you become.

Action Steps:

"How Do I Feel When I Say Yes but Actually Mean No?"

My answer to this question changed a lot for me. When I started asking myself this question and feeling the answer, I noticed that I often said yes when I actually wanted to say no.

If you're like me, you may not be aware of how often you say yes but actually mean no.

Feel free to use your journal for this exercise.

Find a quiet place, take a few deep breaths, and completely relax your body. Close your eyes and ask yourself, "How do I feel when I say yes but actually mean no?"

Then take a few minutes to feel your body with your eyes closed. Try to keep your attention on your body and your breath. Whenever you are distracted, just find your way back to your breath. Let go of any tension and just feel what comes up.

Important: There is no right or wrong here. If you don't feel anything, that's okay. Often the answers to the questions you ask will come later. The more present you are in your daily life, the more you are ready to receive the answer, and the more likely you are to notice when it appears.

You may repeat this exercise several times if you feel that it helps you to find the answer.

Also, after feeling what comes up for a few minutes, take your journal and let the writing flow. Often this is an easier way to find the answer. Whatever wants to come out onto the paper, let it flow. Just write freely from your soul.

Trust the process and have the patience that you will find the answer.

The more I grappled with this question, the more I felt in my body that I was agreeing to something I didn't want to do. I was distracted on the outside, and thus often I didn't notice that I was acting in a way to please my counterpart, even though I actually wanted something else. Asking myself this question has helped me to better inhabit my body. It has helped me to be more with myself, in my power, and to listen to my intuition. This is my goal for you with *Nourish Yourself,* that you will find out more about yourself and your body through every little task and every line. I also hope that you also find your power, radiate your light to the outside world, and learn to listen to your intuition

"How Does My Body Feel When It Is Stressed?"

I deliberately did not include this question with action step 1. If you already know your body better, you can do action steps 1 and 2 together. You can ask yourself both questions and feel what emerges. The important thing with regard to everything within these pages is that it feels right for you.

I have deliberately separated the questions so that you can take your time to feel into both questions separately. You may find that similar answers come up from within your body. It may also be, as mentioned in step 1, that nothing comes, and the answer arrives later, quite unexpectedly. The two exercises are here to help you get more into your body and unleash your power. It's not about you having to *feel* something extreme. I, for example, often just feel a lightness. This lightness tells me that something is right or that I am on the right path. Sometimes I just have this *knowing* inside me. Maybe you are familiar with the feeling that emerges when you can't explain something but know it's the right thing to do.

For this step, you can simply repeat action step 1, but ask yourself the following question: "How does my body feel when it is stressed?"

Again, you may write the answer in your journal or just feel the calmness you create for yourself during the exercise. You decide what feels good and right.

The more often you integrate these exercises into your daily life, the more you will notice that you are getting to know yourself and your body better. Your body is always talking to you, and by doing the simple exercises in *Nourish Yourself,* you will get to know its language better and better. You will learn to live in alignment with your body and be in harmony with it, and this, in turn, leads to the fact that your ability to dissolve any resistance. You are allowed to bed receive and create space for everything you invite into your life.

The Power of Mindful Movement

In my opinion, to release tension or improve my mood, nothing helps more than moving my body to let the energies flow. The important thing is to engage in mindful movement. This doesn't necessarily mean that you have to do yoga. The keyword here is *mindful.* It's about noticing your body, feeling it, and not just pushing it so you can achieve a certain goal.

I wrote at the beginning of this chapter that the energy with which you do something important. This also applies to exercise. The energy you use when doing it is crucial. If you move your body using the energy that it needs to lose weight or build muscle, then you always bring a sessed energy that desperately wants that goal to be achieved. You may achieve your set goal in the process. It may also be that you are doing exactly the opposite.

Before you next start a workout or exercise session, take a few deep breaths in and out and connect with your body for a moment. Focus your attention on your inner self and feel the intention. What energy do you start your workout with?

The key is to feel your body, nourish it, and always focus on your breath. Allow yourself to take short breaks every now and then.

Feel your breath, let it flow, and notice how your body feels. This way you let your energies flow. And the more you connect with your breath, the more you feel yourself and your body.

The Power of Silence–the Magic Sixty

When was the last time you just lay or sat there and did nothing but notice your breath?

When I became aware of how powerful silence really is, how relaxing and magical it is, I made it my daily ritual just to sit there for sixty seconds and notice and feel the silence. This was the moment I created my magic sixty seconds. I do practice it several times a day. Whenever I need a moment, whenever I need some space, I simply sit there for sixty seconds and listen to the silence and be in the present moment.

Surely everyone can set aside sixty seconds from their busy lives. And I always say, those who don't have sixty seconds are those who are in greater need of scheduling sixty-second breaks into their daily lives.

Sixty seconds of just observing silence and listening is an absolute game-changer. I can't recommend enough that you incorporate these magical sixty seconds into your life.

Why sixty seconds?

For some of us, having to sit still for long periods of time is very challenging. It's perfectly normal for our minds to wander during meditation. We have countless thoughts floating in our heads every day, and these don't just disappear when we want to meditate in silence. Others say to themselves that they would like to meditate but can't find the time. Then there are those for whom meditation is not feasible for some other reason.

Sitting quietly for sixty seconds can be done by those who are afraid of their thoughts and therefore are afraid to meditate. Taking sixty seconds to sit quietly is also for those who think they have no time.

Focusing on yourself and your breath for sixty seconds can give you a new perspective at any time. You relax, you bring your attention to yourself, and you are no longer distracted by whatever is outside you. These sixty seconds allow your breath to become calmer and help you find answers. Whenever you are stuck, whenever something seems hopeless, dedicate yourself to the magic sixty. When I am stuck, I take a step back, breathe deep, find myself, and receive the answer.

You can repeat the magic sixty as many times as you like. You can do it several times a day, like me, or you can enjoy the silence for longer than sixty seconds. All you have to do is relax and focus on your breath. Whenever you notice that you are unable to stay focused on your breath, try to count the breaths, or notice and feel your body while breathing. The goal is to be with and stay with yourself. It is about bringing your attention from the outside to the inside. Whenever you seem overwhelmed in your everyday life, the magic sixty will help you to focus on yourself and what is important. I am a big fan of this exercise. It's very simple and very powerful, and you don't feel bad about doing it. Unwith having set out to do something big and being unable to make it happen, you don't need a lot of time or any resources for the sixty seconds. You can implement it in the midst of many people, on the train, or wherever you feel like it.

You might be saying to yourself, *It's not quite on the train or when I'm around a lot of people.* The point of this exercise is to find the silence within you. You may have heard that you can meditate anywhere. It is the same with the magic sixty—it can be done anywhere. The point is that you find the silence within yourself. Whenever you are overwhelmed or stuck on the outside, you can focus on your inner self. Through this small exercise, you learn how to trust in yourself, and how to stay in your center. You achieve more balance in your life, and you strengthen not only your intuition but also your confidence and self-esteem.

Back to You–Basic Breathing Exercise

Your breath controls your inner state. Whenever you breathe quickly and shallowly, you are experiencing stress and tension. Whenever your breath is deep and slow, you are relaxed, and the tension is allowed to release. It is important to connect with your breath every day. It shows you your state. It shows you if you are tense and stressed or if you are in a relaxed state. It is important to create a balance. Whenever you feel that your breath is too fast and shallow, take a moment and focus your attention on your breath.

I have a wonderful breathing exercise for you. It's effective, and it helps you relax and maintain focus. Whenever you feel that you need more balance, take a few minutes and do this exercise. Not only is it simple and doable for everyone, but also you can incorporate it into your daily routine anytime, whenever necessary, whether before an important speech, in the evening to end the day, in the morning to start the day with self-care, or as a small break in your daily routine.

The breathing exercise brings you into the here and now. It lets you come to yourself and causes your attention to automatically turn from the external and return to the internal.

Exercise:

Sit on a chair, on the floor, or on your meditation cushion. It is important that you sit comfortably and if you choose to sit on a chair, that your feet are firmly planted on the floor. Close your eyes slowly and just notice your breath at the beginning. Take a few deep breaths. Feel how your attention slowly turns inward and your tension is released. Let your shoulders relax and allow your hands to rest very loosely on your knees. When you are ready, inhale deeply and count to four silently. Then exhale again and count to four again. Repeat this for ten rounds. On each inhalation, count to four silently, and on each exhalation do the same. When you have done the ten rounds, remain seated with your eyes closed. Let your breath flow at its normal pace as you take a moment to reflect. Consciously feel how you feel inside and be aware of your body. When you are ready, slowly open your eyes.

2.6 **The power of journaling.**

Each of us has different preferences. Some love journaling, whereas for others it is a foreign concept. Whatever the case may be for you, I would like to say a few words about journaling.

Journaling, as well as meditation, brings countless benefits. Nowadays, many studies have shown how journal writing is good for physical health and mental well-being.

I have given journaling a place in *Nourish Yourself* primarily for one reason: it can help you to connect to yourself. The whole of *Nourish Yourself* is basically a guide to taking care of yourself, connecting with your body—loving it, respecting it, and nurturing it—not only to strengthen your intuition and come into your power but also to bring your inner light outward. The purpose of *Nourish*

Yourself is to teach you to be with yourself, to live in the now, to embrace the moment, whatever the moment has to give you, and to write your book, your chapters, here on earth, as you are meant and as you want to write them.

Our daily lives are packed. Everything in our society today points to speed, doing, and competition. This can be very challenging and overwhelming, and it's easy to lose track of everything.

Journaling can be a great support here. By sorting your thoughts and writing them down, placing them on the blank page, you empty your cluttered mind. When you write in a journal, you free yourself from your burden and make room for something new. It can be very liberating simply to write down your thoughts. You may also gain access to your subconscious through writing and suddenly discover blockages or negative beliefs that you never knew were there.

Often it helps to write before or after meditation, to have somewhere to place your thoughts and empty your mind. The good thing about keeping a journey is that you do it just for yourself. You don't have to show anyone what you write in your journal; it's just for you. Write in your journal whenever you feel like it and write whatever you like to write. Detach yourself from whatever you like and connect only with yourself and your thoughts. Again, there are no guidelines for how or what to write, how often you should write, or how much time you should spend. Again, see what feels good, what suits you.

Start with five minutes of journal writing. Feel free to set your timer, then just start writing whatever comes to your mind. It doesn't matter what you write. It is not an essay. No one controls what you write. Nobody checks if you have formulated the sentences correctly. Enjoy these five minutes of me-time. Enjoy the silence for yourself and let the pen move as your thoughts flow. Whatever you want to put on the paper, let the words find their place.

In the beginning, you may feel strange. It can seem very unfamiliar if you have never written before. Repeat this exercise every day if possible. If it is too overwhelming for you to write in your journal every day, start doing it once a week, then increase it to two or three times a week. As with all the other steps in *Nourish Yourself,* it's important to go at your own pace. Feel yourself; find what is right for you. Change leads to change, no matter how small. Walk at your own pace. Walk as many steps per day as feels good to you. The smallest things in your daily life, the smallest change, can lead to the biggest changes ever. Don't judge your pace. And if you fall back into old patterns for a few days, weeks, or months, don't feel bad about it. Start fresh, and then you'll see it gets easier and easier. Believe in yourself, always check your insides to determine what feels good, and follow that good feeling.

Journaling Tips

Especially if you're new to journaling, these tips will help you get started.

1. Create the Right Atmosphere
If you create the right atmosphere for yourself, you'll automatically get into the writing mood. Light some candles, dim the lights, have some music playing in the background. All of this can help you get into the writing mood.

2. Meditate
It can help to meditate beforehand. When you meditate before journaling, you create space and calmness in your body so it can

receive. Whatever wants to come up during meditation, write about it so you can process the emotions properly.

3. Create Stillness

If you don't want to meditate before writing, or if you don't have time to meditate, you can just take a few deep breaths to bring stillness to your body. Quietness often works wonders for getting yourself in the writing mood and accessing your inner self.

4. Set a Timer

It can also be helpful to set your timer for five minutes, ten minutes, or more. As the time ticks down, let your pen slide across the paper. Just write down whatever emerges until the time is up. No judgments. Just let go and let the pen do the work.

5. Write Randomly

You can also do this exercise with a timer or without a time limit. Maybe you'll feel less pressured and not think that you have to write down everything you think in five or ten minutes. Do whatever feels right; you will find the right place. The important thing is that you find relaxation. Allow your body to relax and let go so that you can access your inner self and receive the message that you are meant to receive.

Writing Exercise:

If you find it difficult to start journaling, do the following exercise to help get you started.

Before you start writing, ask yourself the following questions:
- "How am I doing today?"
- "What am I grateful for today?"
- "What was the best thing I experienced today?"

Answering these simple questions will not only help you get started writing but also will help you focus on positive things. When you ask yourself what you're grateful for, you automatically turn your focus to the positive. Try to think of the little things. Maybe a stranger smiled at you today. Maybe you made someone laugh today. It doesn't have to be something big. Often, we tend to block out the little things. This exercise is designed to help you refrain from doing that.

When you answer the question "How am I doing today?" you connect with your body. You turn your attention from the outside to the inside. How often do you pay attention to others and forget about yourself? This should not happen. A small and simple question can do a great deal. From now on, ask yourself every day how you feel. Write down the answer. Let the pen flow and let the words come out onto the paper.

Just as with the gratitude question, by asking about the best thing that happened to you today, you focus your attention on the positive. It helps you immediately shift away from the negative and toward the positive. I often notice myself thinking that I have not had the best day. Then I ask myself these simple questions, and suddenly I think of countless things I am grateful for or that were among the best things about that particular day.

Journaling can help turn the negative into positive. It can lift your spirits and can be very healing and freeing. Just let your feelings flow and put them on paper. Through journaling, you let the energy flow. Instead of pushing down what you feel, you'll allow it to come to the surface. It's enormously important that you allow the feelings to surface, that you let them out. Feel your feelings and process them through journaling. If you don't do this, then the feelings stay in your body, where they get suppressed, so they manifest as negative energy, such as physical pain or sadness.

2.7 **The power of positive affirmation.**

How Do You Talk to Yourself?

Have you ever taken a closer look at how you talk to yourself and how you talk to those around you?

When it comes to self-love, the way you talk to yourself is key.

Before you read on, I invite you to close your eyes for a moment, take a few deep breaths, and observe how you speak to your best friend, your children, and your other loved ones. What words do you use? What do you say to them when they are not feeling well?

After doing that, focus attention on yourself. How do you talk to yourself when you're not doing well, or you've made a mistake? How much time do you take for yourself, and how much time do you spend on your loved ones? Who do you put first?

As always, you can also write the answers in your journal. Take as much time as you need to do this. You can also come back to this exercise whenever you like. Become aware of how you speak to yourself, and what words you choose.

Words are energy; words are a vibration. What energy do you feed yourself every day? What words do you speak to yourself every day?

The more love you give to yourself, the more love you can give to the outside world. If you don't nourish yourself, then you have nothing to pass on. Therefore, it is important not only for you but also for your whole environment that you nourish yourself, that you give yourself love and attention every day.

Self-Talk and Affirmation

I have read about affirmations in books again and again, but I must confess that I have never used them until I came across the work of Louise Hay a few years ago. Louise Hay is, in my opinion, the queen of affirmations. She has written many books, and there are many videos on YouTube of her work on affirmations.

What Is an Affirmation?

An affirmation is a positive phrase that you say to yourself over and over again to reprogram your thoughts and your subconscious mind. It is very important that you never use negative words such as *can't* or *won't* or *never.* Affirmations are always positive.

I invite you today to find your own affirmations, ones that are right for you. The affirmations will help you to transform your negative beliefs about yourself into positive ones. Today, pick the affirmations that will help you empower yourself with positive beliefs, that will give you courage and love, and that will nourish your soul.

If you don't know where exactly to start, which affirmation is right for you, then ask yourself: "What is it that I want to bring into my life? What is it that I would like to achieve?"

For example, if you want to lose weight, write down appropriate affirmations for doing this, affirmations that will positively support you in your endeavor. If you keep telling yourself that you will never lose weight, then this belief will be deeply anchored inside you. By saying you'll never do it, you keep telling yourself that you won't make it, and you feed your energy and subconscious mind with this belief. It's important that you really believe whatever your affirmation is telling you.

Affirmations help you believe in your dream and your goal.

Following are some examples of incorrectly worded affirmations, followed by correctly worded affirmations:

- "I am not stressed." (Write instead: "I am effective [or productive].")
- "I will not eat chocolate today." (Write instead: "I take care of my body" or "I nourish my body with foods my body loves.")

Important: Affirmations always refer to the present. Do not write "I will make a lot of money." This affirmation is in the future. Instead, it is better to write "I have a lot of money."

Write your affirmations on small pieces of paper or in your diary. The important thing is to repeat these affirmations as often as you need to. It is not enough that you say to yourself once "I am successful," or "I am beautiful," or "I am a money magnet." Repetition here is the key. Repeat your affirmations several times each day until they get into your subconscious mind, you believe them 100 percent, and you embody and live your affirmation.

On some days I recite my affirmation every few minutes. On those days I am even more grateful that affirmations exist because they help me find my way out of my negative thoughts. They help me feel good again, and they give me courage and strength.

It is very important that when you repeat your affirmations, you also feel them. I mentioned before those words are energy and each word has its own energy. When you do repeat, your positive affirmation, I invite you to do it by closing your eyes and being really present while you do it. Try to feel the energy of each of your affirmations. Sometimes you might not feel it at all. However, the more you practice it the more you start to believe it and feel it until it manifests into reality.

Now I like you to take a moment and close your eyes. Open them again and read the following questions:

When do you talk bad about yourself?
When do you think badly about yourself?
Where can you change these thoughts into positive ones with the help of positive affirmations?

Take a moment to answer the foregoing questions and pick out the right affirmations that will lead you back into the light when you are facing dark situations. Take your journal and write down what you don't like about yourself, where you judge yourself, and where you talk bad about yourself. Now write down all the negative thoughts you have about yourself. The first step is to be clear about what you think and talk badly about yourself.

The next step is to change your self-talk. Take every bad sentence you wrote about yourself and rewrite it, so it reads as a positive affirmation.

For example, if you wrote "I do not like my body," write simply, "I love my body."

Write the affirmation for each negative sentence and keep the journal with you. Whenever you speak the negative sentences to yourself, say your positive affirmations as many times as necessary to eradicate the negative thought.

There is no one on this planet like yourself.

This is your superpower. Don't forget!

Following are some more affirmations you can use in your daily life:

- "I am beautiful."
- "I am worthy."
- "I am good enough."
- "I am strong."
- "I am powerful."
- "I am a good mother [or wife, or friend, or daughter]."
- "I am always in the right place at the right time."
- "I am guided and supported."
- "I am constantly offered new opportunities."
- "I am productive."
- "I am a money magnet."

2.8 Bring more balance into your daily life.

Our everyday lives are characterized by stress. This points to the fact that our nervous systems are often in a state of stress, and we lack the necessary balance. It is important that our nervous systems become balanced so that we can go through our days in balance.

As already explained in more detail in a previous section, the breath is enormously important for our balance. In addition to our breath contributing to balance, it is also important that our daily routines bring us to balance so that we can go through our days stress-free and full of energy. Women, in particular, tend to give 120 percent every day, no matter the season or time of day.

Why is that actually the case?

I don't have the perfect answer to this. However, it is very important to me, which is why I am writing this section here, that we nourish our bodies, give them gratitude, and live in harmony with them. Each of us has only this one body, and therefore it is important to do good with it. Our bodies work for us every second at full speed so that we can get through the day full of energy. However, if we do not give it what it needs, it cannot give back what we want from it. We are natural beings, and we have a natural rhythm, just like nature has. In spring everything blossoms, in winter, nature takes a break and rests. Animals also live according to their rhythms. Unfortunately, we too often forget that we also have a rhythm. If we don't live in our rhythm, we get out of balance. We have a menstrual rhythm, but also a day and night rhythm.

I used to live by this affirmation: "More is more."

Only when I started to live in harmony with my body and its rhythm did I become really productive and have more energy than ever.

In this section, I give you the opportunity to live more in tune with your body. I offer simple steps to incorporate into your daily routine that will help you go through your day more energized and in tune with your body. With these steps, you'll learn that more is not more and that breaks can actually be productive.

1. The Power of Your Morning Routine

During your morning routine, you set the tone for the day, choosing how you want to rest of the day to be.

Maybe you know this already. There are days when you wake up and you are in a good mood for no reason. However, there are also days when you just want to stay in bed, and you just carry a weird feeling with you. Accordingly, your mood is not good or positive either. I know these days all too well. Just yesterday when I woke up, and even though I'd gone to bed and fallen asleep with very positive thoughts, I had a bad feeling. Sometimes a feeling or mood such as this may be hormonally influenced. Further on, I write a little more in-depth about the menstrual cycle and why it is important to be in balance with it.

But back to the point, each of us has a choice every day. We can surrender to this feeling and give it control and power over us, or we can choose to do the opposite.

With the help of your morning routine, you can redirect your focus. You can choose love and gratitude. You can do something good for yourself, nourish your body with positive things, and move your focus away from negative thoughts and feelings.

Not only do we have a choice in how we start the day, but also, we always have a choice as to how we react to something and how we act in the first place.

The right morning routine can help us and support us in making the rest of the day more positive by lifting our mood and allowing us to start the day with love and gratitude.

All these things have a positive effect not only on the rest of the day, but also on our environment, our work, our family, and yourselves. What energy we radiate, we receive. We always have a choice. We cannot choose what the day holds for us, but we always have a choice in how we respond to what the day brings.

I always carry this thought with me, that I can choose how I do react to something that is happening or that life does present itself. This morning I cut myself twice. The second time I panicked. It bled a lot, and I was immediately caught in the worst-case scenario.

Negative stories came to the surface of my mind right away. I let those stories roll over me for a few minutes. But then I took a few deep breaths. After that, I bandaged my finger and made myself a cup of tea. I knew that I now had a choice in how to respond to what happened. I looked at my to-do list and realized that many of the things I wanted to get done today that made me feel stressed were not that important. Further, I reminded myself that everything happens for a reason. I had cut myself not once, but twice. It was a sign—a sign from the universe showing me to take it easy. More important than the sign was the message behind it. I tend to assume the worst right away. But then I remembered that all that matters is the here and now. I no longer gave the negative stories power over me. I sat down at the computer, answered my emails, and started working through my most important to-dos.

I changed the energy I was putting out and automatically felt my body become calmer. Subsequently, the pain in my finger lessened.

By making time for your morning routine, you are laying the foundation for yourself to become more mindful and present in hectic situations. You also nourish your body with love and self-care. In order to be there for others, you must be there for yourself first and foremost.

How different would your day look if you were to start your day with self-care instead of answering emails or reading negative headlines from the newspaper?

I invite you today to find a morning routine that works for you. You don't have to set aside two hours. Of course, you can if you want to. But just a few minutes can change a lot of things.

I've had my fixed morning routine for years. It's part of my daily routine; it's part of my life. When I don't have much time, I can make my morning routine a little shorter. When I have more time, I enjoy really celebrating my morning routine.

The important thing is to find the right routine for you, including its length and the things you choose to do first in order to start the day at your best and full of energy. Each of us is different, so it's important that you don't compare your routine to a friend's or anyone else's. What is important is that you create a positive morning routine for yourself, one that nourishes you gives you positive energy and helps you walk through the day present and nourished.

There are a few things you should keep in mind when it comes to making sure you find the right morning routine for you. They are as follows:

Ensure There Are No External Distractions

Try to use the time for yourself. Connect with yourself and your body. As soon as you turn your attention to the outside, such as an email or the radio, you lose control. You are distracted, and all your energy is already externally focused. When you start the day with yourself and go within, you create a foundation that gets you through the day. Whenever you need a break during the day, take a deep breath and feel that power and energy you created in the morning. It is there. Whenever you need it, use it to arrive at the moment and connect with your center.

Observe a Few Minutes of Mindfulness

As mentioned earlier, the key to the perfect morning routine is to start your day not with outside things, but with yourself. You can start your day with a wonderful meditation, a breathing exercise, or complete silence. Start your day with a few minutes of mindfulness. Connect with your body. Feel how your body is and how you feel and embrace the moment. Be present. Enjoy the silence and the moment.

A few minutes of mindfulness can help you be more in your power and put you more in balance throughout the day. You may notice that situations that used to easily throw you off track affect you less because you are present and with yourself. Not only does this make you less stressed, but also it helps you be more productive throughout the day because you are more focused and centered.

Start with Something That Brings You Joy and Positively Influences Your Mood

We all have those days when we wake up in a poor mood. If we start the day with joy, then the foundation for a positive day is set.

What is it that you can do first thing in the morning to feel joy? What is it that nourishes you, do you good, and brings you joy?

Joy is energy. It's primarily about nourishing your whole body in the morning with wonderful, positive joyful energy.

When you are asked the question of what activity brings you joy, you have two choices. You can actually start your day with that activity. Maybe you feel pure joy when you read a book. Maybe you feel pure joy when you drink your coffee. Maybe you're reading this right now and you're saying to yourself, *I don't get any joy out of my morning activities.* You might be thinking that everything that brings you joy doesn't fit into your routine in the morning because (a) you don't have time or (b) they are simply things that are not feasible in the morning.

If these two points are indeed true, then you should definitely rethink your priorities. How do you set your daily priorities? In order to achieve your goal, you must implement certain practices. You can't expect to become a marathon runner if you never train for it. Do you want to bring more balance into your day? If the answer is yes, then you need to implement certain practices. In order for you to reshape your day, and especially your morning routine, you need to create a window of time for doing so. As I mentioned before, I don't have the same amount of time each day for my morning routine. However, I know that without it, I am only half balanced, partially nourished, and partially stressed, so my chance of being stressed and overwhelmed for the rest of the day is much greater. This would in turn affect my environment, especially my family, and also my work. When I perform my morning routine, I am doing something good not only for myself but also for my whole environment. My morning routine has therefore become an integral part of my day and vital to my whole being. I make time for it every day, be it even just a few minutes.

Is your long-term goal to find more balance in your everyday life so that you can achieve your goals in the long run and become more focused? If so, then close your eyes for a moment and search your feelings to discover what you can do in the morning to bring yourself joy and help lay the foundation for a positive and productive day. If it is difficult for you to answer this question, then trust that the answer will find you.

Have you found the answer to the question and are having a hard time implementing it? Do you lack space in your home for implementation? Or are you missing something else that is preventing you from implementing it?

As mentioned earlier, joy is nothing more than a form of energy. This point is about stepping into the day with positive energy so that you lay the foundation for a successful day. Whatever the day will bring, the likelihood that you will draw positive things into it increases many times over if you are already positively nourishing your whole body and positively tuning your whole being in the morning.

You can start your day with something that brings you joy, or you may choose to take a few minutes, close your eyes, and visualize that which causes you to feel joy. Let your imagination run wild. Maybe you are at the beach or driving down the street in a Ferrari. The important thing is the joy you feel. Feel the joy intensely with every cell of your body. Feel what it is like when you are on the beach or wherever else you want to be. Stay as long as you like. Feel the feelings deep within and nourish every cell of your body with this wonderful, joyful energy. Feel your mood change instantly and, with it, your whole being. You are laying the foundation not only for the day, but also for your future.

Practice Mindful Movement

The human body holds on to a great deal of negative energy. In order to release everything, you no longer want to carry with you, you must let the energy flow. Movement is the perfect solution for this. With mindful movement, you not only connect to your body but also let the energy flow. The body relaxes and is able to let go in the process.

A little stretching or a few minutes of movement is all it takes to get the energy flowing. Take a walk in nature, do some yoga, stretch, or do whatever you like to move your body. There is no right or wrong here. The point is to allow the body to relax and the energies to flow.

Eat a Nourishing Breakfast

In chapter 3, you will learn more about energy and food. Eating the right breakfast will help you start the day full of energy. With a healthy, nourishing breakfast, you not only do something good for your body but also influence your mood positively.

The Right Breakfast

How often do we hear or read that breakfast is the most important meal of the day? Every meal is important. However, I subscribe to this idea 100 percent. But not that I think you should eat breakfast like a king.

Daily breakfast should provide you with energy, not rob you of it. Breakfast should nourish your body and help you start the day full of energy.

As mentioned in chapter 3, food is a form of energy for the body. It is therefore important that you give your body the right form of energy to get through the day optimally. If your digestion is not functioning optimally, then it robs you of strength and energy. Valuable energy is lost to you that you could otherwise be using for many things.

I myself have too often followed a diet plan. For years I was looking for the right diet for me. Today I know that what is right for me is not necessarily right for you. You'll find some breakfast recipes in chapter 7. But this doesn't mean that from now on, you should eat only one of these recipes in the morning. Take the recipes as inspiration. If you have yet to find the right breakfast for you, take your time. Start each day with new breakfast, then write down how you feel after eating it. Does it fill you up? Does it give you energy? Does it help your digestion? Food can rob the body of so much precious energy. To find the right food for you that will give you what you need in the morning to get the best start to your day.

There are a few things you should keep in mind when it comes to eating the right breakfast:

Eat When You Are Hungry

Personally, I cannot go without breakfast. There are people, my husband, for example, who don't need breakfast. Maybe you are one of these people, even if you have always thought that breakfast is the most important meal of the day.

I believe that the body signals us when it needs something to eat. If we are not hungry, then there is likely a reason for that. We all have different digestion; some digest good faster than others and therefore need to eat more because they get hungry again sooner.

If you listen to your body, then you know when you are hungry. Then you learn to eat when you feel hungry.

Eat a Light Breakfast

As mentioned before, you may have heard that breakfast is the most important meal of the day, or that you should eat breakfast like an emperor and dinner like a beggar. I am not suggesting that you cut your breakfast portion in half. As I mentioned earlier, food is a form of energy. So, if you start the day by eating heavy foods, you are robbed of valuable energy for the day. Your digestion will be busy operating at full speed, causing you to lose the energy you need for everyday life.

Eat a Nourishing Breakfast

Choosing the right breakfast for your body gives you not only a lot of energy but also important nutrients. In the morning, with an empty stomach, the body can absorb food better than at other times during the day. The body is not busy digesting lunch or an afternoon snack. All its attention belongs to the first bite you take. Therefore, it is recommended that you start the day with a healthy, nourishing healthy breakfast such as green juice or a green smoothie. The body can focus 100 percent on the green leafy vegetables, which are among the most nutrient-dense vegetables and provide the body with many valuable minerals and vitamins, fiber, and of course lots of energy for the day.

In the next chapter, you will find wonderful breakfast recipes. They are all very easy to prepare, and they nourish your body, satisfy your hunger, and support your digestion.

2. Winding Down with Your Evening Routine

For more balance in everyday life, besides a morning routine, it is important to have an evening routine. Unfortunately, most of us have completely forgotten how to live in harmony with nature. In the past, when it used to get dark, we would light a few candles, talk, enjoy the evening, and go to bed. Today, we watch countless movies on Netflix in the evening, and instead of our body being able to relax and shut down, we stimulate it with blue light.

We are still natural beings, and it is our destiny to live in harmony with nature. When we don't do so, our bodies become imbalanced, so we get out of balance and are not grounded and centered. This affects our mood, our health, and our whole energy level.

Our bodies need breaks and rest, especially in the evening if we are to start the next day full of energy. Therefore, not only the morning routine but also the evening routine is very important for our balance. Routines are generally important for us. They give us security. We, humans, are creatures of habit. A fixed daily routine gives us stability. Even as babies, we learn to distinguish between day and night. Our mothers help us learn to sleep at night. We also learn to get used to fixed mealtimes. These little things give us security and help us feel safe.

There is no right or wrong when it comes to your evening routine. As mentioned before, we are each unique and often are very different from one another. For some, the perfect evening routine is taking a bath; for others, it's drinking a cup of tea and reading a good book.

To help you find the routine that's right for you, I've provided a few tips. These tips are nothing more than guidelines. Take what works for you, and step by step create the right and nourishing evening routine that will help you balance your body, recover, and shut down.

Eat a Healthy Dinner at the Right Time

Maybe you're like me on this one. Every time I go out and eat a little more than usual, I have trouble falling asleep. So the body may digest dinner optimally and get restful sleep, it is recommended that you eat no food for two to three hours before going to bed. This will give your body the time it needs to digest your dinner optimally.

In chapter 7, you will find some recipes for healthy and nourishing foods. The recipes are not only simple but also quick to prepare, and most of the time you can cook them in double quantity, so you need only to heat up the meal for the next day.

In the next section, you will find more detailed information about mindfulness in the kitchen and at mealtime. This will help you end the evening with the right dinner and atmosphere.

Find Peace—No Distractions

The evening is the time for darkness, quiet, and stillness. If you are not aware of what gives you this feeling, I recommend you take your journal and do some soul-searching. What things give you the feeling of peace and stillness? Maybe a wonderful meditation session? Reading a book? Maybe you find peace when you stretch your body or when you take a bath? Take your time for this exercise and write down everything that comes to your mind. When you're done, close your eyes and concentrate on what you feel inside. Which of these things nourish your body? Which of these thigivesgive it peace and stillness? Maybe it will help you to imagine yourself doing these things. What feeling comes up when you imagine yourself doing any of the things you wrote about? As mentioned, many times before, it's about the feeling behind you do. Stillness is nothing more than a form of energy. Silence is a form of energy, as is darkness. It's about creating the energy of stillness in your body so that it knows that evening has come. It is allowed to review the day, relax, and shut down.

Create the Proper Lighting

There is a reason why the day comes with light, and it gets dark in the evening. To best signal to your body that evening has come, the time to come down, it is important to dim the lights. Maybe you'd like to light a few candles or dim your lamps in your apartment or house. Create a wonderful atmosphere with lights that will help you relax and then find optimal sleep.

Have a Fixed Bedtime

As mentioned before, we humans are creatures of habit. The body carries an internal clock inside. In order for this to function optimally, you should have a fixed bedtime.

You should also rise at the same time each morning. Find the optimal balance for you.

3. How to Balance through the Different Seasons

The answer to how you can achieve more balance in your daily life is simple: live in harmony with nature—starting with your morning routine, moving through your evening routine, and traveling into each season. The trees and flowers in nature have their annual rhythms. This is also true for us humans. Unfortunately, this rhythm has been completely lost to most of us. It does not take much time or effort to get back into this rhythm. A few small things in everyday life can help you to adjust your rhythm to that of the seasons and thus find more balance and energy.

Following are a few tips that you can use to find and maintain your balance throughout the year:

Eat Seasonally

Not only do we have twenty-four-hour access to food today, but also, we are able to get out-of-season fruits and vegetables throughout the year. As a result, we often forget which foods are in season. For example, summertime is berry season; pumpkins are harvested in fall, and parsnips are available in wintertime. Now you don't have to print out a seasonal calendar and hang it up, although you can if you want to. Just being a little more mindful when you are grocery shopping is all it takes. In the supermarket, you will usually see a sign that shows if something is in season or where the food comes from. You can use this as a guide.

If you listen to your body, you will discover that it demands different meals in winter than it does in summer. I myself love to enjoy a big salad with delicious toppings in the summer. In winter, my body demands warm food. The reason for the latter is obvious: it is cold outside, the nights are long, and the body craves warmth and comfort. During the colder seasons, it is therefore recommended that you enjoy stews and soups that nourish you and warm you from the inside. During the warmer months, the best nourishment for the body is a tasty salad or generally more raw vegetables. Of course, as mentioned many times in *Nourish Yourself*, it is important that everyone listen to their body's own needs. People who get colder much faster generally need more warm cooked meals than those who tend to produce body heat more easily.

If you listen to your body and interpret the signals correctly, you will always find what is right for you. With *Nourish Yourself*, you have help to know your body better and understand it.

Get Ready for the Dark Season

Autumn invites you to settle in at home. The days slowly become shorter and colder, the nights, longer. Nature is preparing for winter, the time of rest. Soon the white blanket falls from the sky, and so follows hibernation for some animals and also plants. Of course, this is not true for us. We can't hole up all the time, yet the darker time of the year invites us to settle in at home. We begin spending more time at home. Create an atmosphere at home that nourishes you and does you good. Perhaps add a few candles and the appropriate decoration. Again, what you choose is very individual. The point is that you find a balance. By creating a relaxing atmosphere in your home, you create a place of retreat, a place where your batteries are recharged. This is important for the whole year, but it is even more important for the colder and darker seasons, as you tend to be outside less and therefore have less sunlight to nourish you, which can also affect hormones and mood.

Adapt Your Exercise to Nature

As mentioned in the previous point, the darker time of the year generally means less time spent outside and more spent inside. However, a daily exercise routine is still very important. So, how can you move your body on a daily basis? What does your body need in the winter, and what exercise does it love in the summer? It may be that you jog or swim a lot in the summer. Maybe in winter, you find an indoor swimming pool instead of the lake. Maybe you visit the yoga studio around the corner in the winter instead of jogging in the woods. Maybe you go for a wonderful walk in the snow. Daily exercise is important for health and well-being.

4. Daily Breaks

Daily breaks are tremendously important for optimal balance. This is important to keep the nervous system in balance. We tend to always be *doing*. At the same time, it is important to switch to *being* from time to time. Taking breaks does not mean being lazy. These little breaks are enormously important for productivity. They help us stay focused. This focus in turn helps us to be productive. Just a few minutes can be enough and be a real game-changer. Take a few small timeouts every day. Not only will you support your health and keep your nervous system in balance, but also, you'll stay more focused and concentrated, which means you'll have more energy and be more productive throughout the day.

I like to think of it as the yin and yang. It takes both things for the whole thing to work. One side alone is not complete. You too need two sides to be whole. These two sides are reflected as doing and being. The balance of the two sides is crucial. If you are too much in doing, you need to balance yourself by being.

5. Never Skip Self-Care

I can't stress this enough: *never, ever skip self-care*. In order for you to be there for others, in order for you to completely take care of others, it is essential that you take care of yourself. Your soul needs nourishment, soul food. Things will not go well if you are always there only for others, completely forgetting yourself. If you neglect yourself, you will eventually get out of balance. Self-care is enormously important for balance. It not only nourishes you but also gives you something to pass on. You have nourishment to give to others, such as your loved ones.

2.9 I love my body and my body loves me.

If you ask me, self-care and self-love is the basis of everything. It affects every area of one's life.

For the past few years, the concept of self-care has been more present than ever. I have the feeling that everywhere you look, people are talking about self-care. Of course, this is a good thing, as self-care, in my opinion, along with self-love, is the foundation for everything.

Whereas it is a good thing to take time to have a cup of tea or do something good for yourself, true self-love and self-care, to me, go deeper. It's about loving yourself and accepting yourself for who you are. It's about going deeper, noticing the feelings and why they come up. It's about recognizing where you are blocked and why you are afraid. It's about not comparing yourself but living your power, being who you are.

I hope with the tools I share in this section you will find what you need to make self-care a part of your life. However, self-care without self-love is only half of the whole in my opinion. If you don't love yourself wholeheartedly, then any time you make for yourself will do only a partial job. Don't get me wrong, time for yourself is hugely important. It helps you switch off; it nourishes you and gives you energy. But if self-love is missing, then your glass is only half full.

I have started to remind myself daily of the following mantra: "I love my body and my body loves me."

This affirmation has helped me not only to be more in my body but also to realize what my body needs. It is a small mantra that made and still makes an enormous impact on me. Whenever I get a little off track (and yes, I have bad days or even bad periods in my life), this mantra brings me back like no other. It reminds me how important my body is to me, also reminding me that I have only this one body and that I want to do good for it.

We women especially tend to compare ourselves and often find something wrong with our bodies. None of us is perfect, and that's a good thing. We are unique. It's the little flaws that make someone truly beautiful if you ask me. Beauty for me comes from within. Beauty comes from the heart.

Your body is beautiful the way it is. It loves you, and today I invite you to love your body back.

Whenever you need it, repeat the affirmation: "I love my body and my body loves me."

Maybe you like to meditate with this it, like me. I sit on my meditation cushion, close my eyes, take a few deep breaths, and then silently repeat "I love my body and my body loves me". After a few minutes, it never fails to warm my heart and give me love for my being and my body.

Try it yourself. Sit in a quiet place, either on your meditation cushion, on the floor, or on a chair. Close your eyes and breathe in and out slowly. Feel your breath, be aware of your body, and then silently repeat: "I love my body and my body loves me."

Repeat it as long as necessary. When you are ready, slowly come back into your body. Notice again your breath going in and out, then slowly open your eyes.

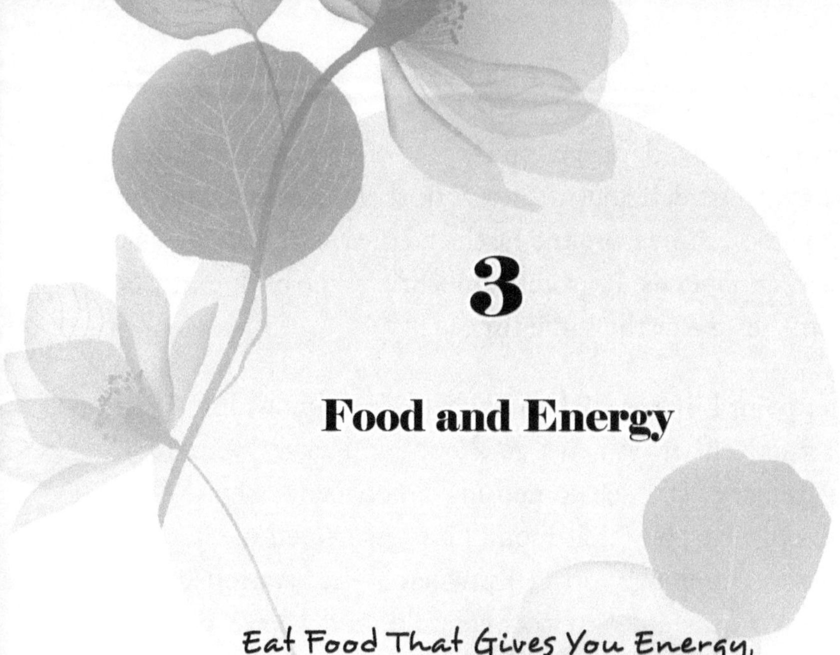

3

Food and Energy

Just as everything else is energy, our diet, the foods we eat, is also a form of energy.

Depending on what foods you choose the energy in your body can change. With my dietary changes, I have noticed how my consciousness has changed when it comes to food. I have learned what really gives me energy, what is good for me, and what is not.

We are all individuals, so we each have different needs and different preferences. What is right for some can be the exact opposite for others. Therefore, nothing is right or wrong.

My personal mantras when it comes to nutrition are "Back to basics" and "Less is more."

A meal doesn't always need bells and whistles to be good and satisfying. Consider that the digestive system often becomes overwhelmed when one eats too many different components together. That's why I always cook and create my recipes with the motto "Less is more." I also like to remember how my grandmother cooked for her family. She often chose potatoes and created the most delicious dishes with them. Potatoes, including sweet potatoes, come from the earth and give us grounding energy. I love eating potatoes. It grounds me, brings me back to my body, and nourishes me at the same time.

Another point I like to stick to is what I don't know, my digestion doesn't know either. When I go shopping, I read the ingredients on the package. If I see something I don't understand or don't recognize, I don't buy that food. This has helped me a lot when it comes to shopping, especially when I first started changing my diet. My kids are now six years old, and I have passed this technique on to them. I simply ask them if they absolutely want something that is a convenience food and not really nutritious or healthy, if their stomachs will recognize the ingredients in that food.

Another rule I have set for myself: Is don't say no.

If we forbid ourselves something or say no to something, such as chocolate, for example, the consequence is that our body will want it even more. That's how it is with bans in general. We "cannot" have something, so the consequence is that we want it all the more. This is best illustrated by little children. As we know, if you tell them no, it doesn't help very much. They still want whatever it is they're asking for, and after hearing no, they only want it more.

For me, it's all about balance. It's what I eat most of the time that counts, not what I eat once in a while. The important thing is to be intentional about eating my chocolate cake. Be present; enjoy it to the fullest. We digest the feelings we feel when we eat just as much as we digest the food itself. How do you think the body feels when it gets that piece of chocolate cake and enjoys it 100 hundred percent? On the other hand, how does the body feel to eat that piece of chocolate cake along with feeling regret or stress?

When you indulge in a piece of chocolate cake, indulge to the fullest. Enjoy it; be present with it. Too often we eat unconsciously, at work, on the go, or in front of the TV. Our minds are not on the food, which leads to eating too fast, not chewing enough, and even overeating.

As with everything, it is important to be present when eating. Ask your body if it is even hungry, what is it asking for, and why it is asking for it. The more you listen to your body, the more you are able to determine when you are actually hungry and when you are full. This way you won't run the risk of overeating or unconsciously eating something that your body doesn't want and hasn't asked for.

We are natural beings, which means we need food that has not been processed but comes from nature. Therefore, it is important to choose natural fresh foods. Cooking doesn't have to be time-consuming, and it doesn't have to be complicated. In chapter 7, I share a few of my recipes that are easy to replicate and also very quick to make. Many of us spend a good deal of time on social media these days, so for those who think they don't have time to cook and for those who prefer to choose processed convenience foods, think about your day, including where can you set aside time for yourself and for cooking. After all, you are doing something good for yourself and your body when you cook yourself a meal. Cooking is love. In the following sections, I go into more detail about why mindfulness is very important when it comes to eating and cooking.

3.1 **Mindfulness about food.**

The more we are in our power, the more present we are, and so the more natural and easier it is when it comes to our nutrition. We automatically feel what is good for us. We eat when we are hungry and nourish our bodies with unprocessed food, giving them the love and attention, they need.

Every day, we waste so much energy on outside concerns. We get distracted, we are energetically drained, and on top of that, we hardly take time for our food. How often do I hear, "I quickly eat something on the way to the office" or "I don't take a lunch break, just quickly eat a sandwich at the computer"?

The mothers give all their attention to their dear children, and so often they end up only eating their little ones' leftovers. They cook for their loved ones, spend time doing good for them, nourish them with food and their love, but too often forget to nourish themselves and give themselves the attention they deserve.

How often do you find yourself making time for the gym or sports in general but not making time for the meal before or after, and instead just grabbing a quick bar or power drink?

We spend so much money on expensive creams, clothes, jewelry, and other material things, but when it comes to food, too often we take the fast and therefore unhealthy way by choosing a sandwich on the go, not taking time to cook fresh food at all.

We live in a society that is dominated by hecticness. For us, being successful means that we have to work a lot. We have the feeling of being important when we have a lot to do and little time for ourselves. People who are at home and have no appointments are not successful in our minds. In addition, everything has become very fast-paced.

We live in a world dominated by fast-moving, hectic energy. It is very important to find a balance. To get this balance, we must ground ourselves, rest, and relax. Self-care rituals such as meditation, writing in a diary, taking a bath, or going into nature can create just the right balance to hectic everyday life.

We also often forget that the food we eat is energy. But it's not just the food on the plate that we eat; everything around it is energy too. Perhaps you have heard the phrase "Everything is energy." Therefore, it stands to reason that everything around food is nothing but energy.

Our bodies absorb the food we give them, but we must not forget that our bodies also absorb the energy of how we eat our food, how it was cooked, and what thoughts, feelings, and emotions we had in the process. The body absorbs all of that. So, again, it digests the food that it gets and everything around it. Therefore, often the reason for flatulence, constipation, or discomfort is not the food itself, but rather everything around it. Stress, for example, can play a big role when it comes to digestion.

Therefore, it is important for your well-being to practice mindfulness around the topic of food. Following you will find some action steps for inviting more mindfulness into your life when it comes to food:

Action Steps Relating to Food and Mindfulness:

Ask yourself: "What intention do I have for cooking this meal?"

The next time you are in the kitchen preparing food for yourself, your family, or other loved ones, take a moment.

How often do you stand in the kitchen preparing a meal stressed out, completely famished, and tired? If you're like me, then you use your time for many things. In the process, the preparation of the meal often comes up short. Yet this time is enormously important and should be a priority. Meals nourish the body so that it gets energy.

You have only this one body, so you should take care of it. With the right choice of food, you help your body to give you valuable energy.

The energy with which you prepare your meal is just as crucial as the choice of food. You may be aware that a ready-to-eat pizza is not the best choice for a balanced dinner. Are you also aware that the energy with which you prepare your meal plays an important role? Your body digests not only the food you eat. The energy with which you approach eating something is equally absorbed by your body.

Before you go into the kitchen next time and cook yourself a meal, take a moment to connect with your body and check-in with yourself. How are you feeling today? Are you stressed or exhausted, or are you looking forward to cooking something? Are you cooking with love or because you have to? What is your intention for finding your way into the kitchen?

In chapter 4, about spirituality, I write about how everything is energy. The emotion with which you prepare our meal is another form of energy. This energy transfers to your food. It flows into your meal.

From now on, just before going to the kitchen, feel your inner self for a moment. Take a few deep breaths and detach yourself from your negative thoughts and emotions. Focus completely on preparing a delicious, nourishing meal for yourself or your loved ones, and be complete with yourself. Cook with love and in your own presence. This energy will transfer to your food and ultimately nourish every cell in your body.

How Do You Want Your Food to Make You Feel?

The food we eat is a form of energy. Not every food automatically provides us with the same energy. Fresh, unprocessed foods provide our bodies with a different form of energy than processed foods do.

Nowadays we take far too little time for our food, be it for the preparation or for the food itself. We tend to forget that what we eat every day provides us with our daily energy.

When we take a moment to ask ourselves how we want our food to make us feel, we bring our attention to the here and now. We draw attention to ourselves with this question.

If you already ask yourself daily how you want your food to make you feel, then the probability that you will choose food that nourishes you, your body, and your whole being and provides you with a lot of positive energy is automatically increased.

With this simple question, you automatically bring yourself and your body into the now. You feel your body and are willing to do something good for yourself.

It doesn't take much effort or time. One question, one small moment, is enough to be more mindful, listen to your body, and to something good for it and yourself.

You can change your whole being with the help of food. I personally love to eat grounding foods in the evening, such as potatoes or carrots—vegetables that are easy to digest, nourishing, and filling and that come from the earth. Vegetables from the earth automatically give the body grounding energy. Young foods such as sprouts, for example, give the body boyish energy. A few sprouts on your avocado toast can be wonderful for your body.

It is important to be aware when asking how you want your food to make you feel that you are not using food to suppress or satiate your feelings. How often do we not really enjoy the chocolate or the cake, but try to suppress something in the process of eating it? Later in this section, I go into the topic of feelings and food in more detail.

Cook with Love—Back to Basics

I used to think, not only in sports or at work, but in many cases, that more was more. I also had this belief that I was not good at cooking. I always thought I had to cook fancy foods and that more was more. I was able to shed this belief a few years ago, and today I invite you to do the same.

Since I've been cooking according to the "Back to basics" mantra, not only do I save time, but also my digestion really thanks me. It may seem wonderful to have ten or more foods and ingredients on your plate. All of these foods and ingredients enter the digestive tract at the same time, so it now has the task of digesting everything at once. This is a lot of work. Therefore, it may well be that something that normally causes no digestive difficulties suddenly leads to bloating or poor digestion. The reason is quite simple: the digestive system is overwhelmed by the sumptuous meal. Therefore, I recommended that you put less on your plate and eat mindfully so that your digestion is supported in the process.

I like to recall how my grandmother cooked for me when I was little. Her meals were made with love and were very simple in design. I try to cook the same way for myself and my family today. Simple meals cooked with love also bring loving and nourishing energy to the body. During my training as an integrative nutrition health coach at IIN in New York (https://www.integrativenutrition.com/), I learned the importance of cooking with the vitamin L. *L* is for "love." I have already mentioned that everything is energy. (In chapter 4, about spirituality, I write about this in more detail.) So it is with vitamin L. Whoever cooks with love puts love on the plate, and this love may be absorbed along with the food by the body. Whoever reaches for the wooden spoon stressed, tired, or angry thus transfers this energy to the plate and, further, to others or to oneself.

Of course, when it comes to the act of cooking, mindfulness is a must. Therefore, I offer a few tips for how you can bring more mindfulness to your cooking.

How to Achieve Mindfulness while Cooking:

<u>Always Cook with Love</u>

As I mentioned already, the energy you have while you cook for yourself or your loved ones is very important as this energy is automatically transmitted to the food, so it ends up in the body. The digestive system does so much more than just digesting the food you eat. The energy that accompanies your food is digested by your body too.

Cook with the Right Intention

What is your intention while you cook your food? Do like to nourish yourself and your body with a lovely meal? Are you actually stressed as you have to cook for yourself or even your family and you would rather be doing something else?

Get clear on the intention behind your cooking. This intention is energy too, and you automatically bring that energy to your food.

As I mentioned several times, everything is energy; therefore, the way you cook, the intention behind it, is energy too.

Your body is your vehicle, and it needs attention and fuel to function. You have only this one vehicle. If it ceases to function, you won't get a new one.

Choose a Positive Affirmation while You Cook Your Dinner

As I mentioned in the previous chapter, I love affirmations and they are a big part of my life. By choosing a positive affirmation for yourself while you cook, you automatically bring positive energy to your cooking. Cooking is the perfect time to practice positive affirmations. Say your affirmation out loud or listen to a podcast or a video on YouTube while you cook. This could help you not only feel better but also bring positive energy to the food that you put into your body.

Notice Your Energy while You Cook

Before you start cooking, take a moment to breathe deeply and simply check in with yourself. Connect to your body and your energy. Feel your body. You may even want to ask yourself how you feel today.

By just checking in a moment, you not only bring yourself to the present moment but also bring attention to your body. You notice how your body is feeling. You automatically get away from the head, out of thinking mode, and enter feeling mode.

All it takes is just a moment of presence, which can create a big shift in your being, bring you away from thinking, and return you to just being.

Breathe Deeply and Slowly while You Cook so Your Body Feels Relaxed

As I just mentioned, all it takes is just a moment of presence to create a big shift and bring you away from thinking and back to just being.

Your breath is very powerful. All you need to do is simply take a few deep, slow breaths to create a big shift in your body and your whole being. You have the power over yourself and your body. Whenever you feel stressed and overwhelmed, all it takes is a few deep, slow breaths to help you to return to yourself and put your body in a relaxed state. Focus on your breath and you are in the here and now. Focus on your breath and you live in the present moment. The present moment is your weapon because in the present moment, you have access to your inner power.

Have Gratitude for Yourself and Your Body while Cooking

The body works 24/7 at its best capacity. It is natural to us that we can walk, that we breathe, and that have the ability to stay in the kitchen and cook. Take a moment and thank yourself and your body for being healthy, for its ability to be in the kitchen, and for your ability to cook a nice meal for yourself or your loved ones. Don't fall into the trap of taking much for granted and forgetting what a miracle your body is. Start each cooking session by saying a little prayer to yourself and having gratitude for staying in the kitchen and cooking a lovely nourishing meal.

Too often people forget that eating is so much more than simply satisfying the feeling of hunger. As mentioned earlier, too often today, too little time is allotted for eating itself. A quick sandwich to go, a protein shake after a workout, breakfast at the computer, or dinner on the way home—this is everyday life for many of us. Since everything is energy and the body digests according to how we eat, the thoughts and emotions we're having and the activity we're performing, mindfulness while eating is very important. Practice more mindfulness while eating by using the following action steps. Not only will they help you be more aware while you eat your meals, but also, they will support your overall well-being and help you step more mindfully through your day, learning what is good for your body and what is not.

Action Steps for Mindful Eating:

Choose a Quiet Environment

As already asked in this chapter, how many times do you eat on the go? How many times do you not take time to eat or chew? How many times do you eat with distractions, such as your phone, your TV, loud music, or a magazine or book?

Perhaps you have heard the phrase "You are what you eat."

In my opinion, "You are what you digest" would be more appropriate. You can eat as many vegetables and fruits as you want, but your body has to digest these wonderful nourishing foods. If the body does not digest the food properly, then it stays in your system, causing the energy to flow improperly.

This is why mindfulness when eating is so important. How you prepare something, how you chew it, the environment in which you eat your meal—all these things play an important role.

So, the first step in eating your meal is to ensure a conducive environment. The next time you cook something to eat, check in with yourself first. Are you on the go? Are you in a hurry? Are you able to take enough time to chew your food? Are you enjoying your meal? Are you eating in a busy environment with lots of distractions?

Be mindful of your environment while you eat your food. It is important that you take the time to chew your food, so it is digested properly.

Chew Your Food

I never paid much attention to my chewing. But it actually is very important that we chew our food properly. The stomach does not have any teeth to make the food any smaller. Everything that is too big for the digestive system will not be digested properly. So that your digestive system can work at its best and your energy can flow and chew your food properly.

Eat slowly. Take your time while you eat your food. Do not take the next bite until you have swallowed the one in your mouth.

Notice Why You Eat

How do you feel while eating your food? Are you stressed and simply eating some chocolate because your stress level is high? Are you feeling bored, tired, lonely, sad, or angry?

I highly recommend that you check in with yourself before you go and get a treat for yourself.

For many years I would eat based not on my level of hunger but based simply on being bored. Whenever I felt bored, I went to get chocolate or whatever sweets I could find. And it gets worse: I enjoyed these treats while watching some stupid TV show. I was not paying attention to my feelings at all. I was not mindful; I simply ate because I was feeling bored.

The day I noticed this behavior changed everything. Food is energy for the body. Food is not there to satisfy feelings. When you are bored, go outside, move around, play a game, or read a book—whatever alleviates your boredom. Food isn't made to take the edge off boredom. You alone can distract yourself and ensure you stop being bored.

When you're stressed, angry, or even sad, again, food is not the solution. It only causes you to suppress your feelings. It takes a lot of energy to allow your feelings to surface, and that's not always very easy to do. Nevertheless, when you try to satisfy your feelings with food, they stay in your body—and sooner or later they come to the surface. You do nothing more than suppress your feelings when you resort to food instead of feeling those feelings. It is important to feel your feelings so that your energy can flow instead of staying blocked in your body. The energy that is blocked in the body is toxic energy. This energy may be eliminated by keeping it flowing.

Nourish Yourself offers support and suggestions to keep your energy flowing. The suggestions herein, if implemented, help you to go through your day more mindfully, enabling you to recognize your feelings, to feel them, and thus to let the energy flow. That way, you automatically practice being nonresistance. Being in a state of nonresistance means you will receive *abundance*. You are in a state where you can receive everything that the universe has in store for you. Everything that is meant to come into your life will flow easily into your life. You allow it as you resist nothing and let the energy move through you and flow.

Practice Being Grateful

Being grateful for your food brings abundance to your plate and your body. When you say that you are thankful for your food, you nourish your food with love, and this love enters your body and flows through you.

You can simply say a little prayer before eating, or you can share with loved ones at the table what you are for grateful today.

I play this game every day with my kids. We have turned practicing being grateful into a little game. Everyone shares at the table what they are grateful for. We are also each share what our favorite moment of the day was. Doing this automatically causes the mind to remember the positive things about the day. It lifts one's mood and energy to focus on the positive rather than the negative.

Practice Being Mindful in Everyday Life

Morning

Start your day with a morning routine that nourishes you and causes you to be mindful.

Your morning routine might look like this: drink warm water with lemon, meditate, journal, stretch or do a small workout, and eat a nourishing breakfast (find some breakfast recipes in chapter 7).

In section 2.8, you will find more ideas on creating a morning routine that helps you start your day nourished and mindful.

During the Day

Take time for small breaks every now and then. Focus on your breath—breathe in and out—and connect with your body.

It is important to keep your nervous system in balance. Whenever you feel that you are stressed or you lose perspective, take a step back and observe the situation from the outside, like a third person. Focus all your attention on your internals. Let go of the thoughts in your head and focus on your center. Notice your breath and feel it as you inhale and exhale deeply.

It takes only a few seconds or a few minutes to realign your focus, move away from stress, and recenter yourself.

Evening

The evening is the time to slowly prepare the body for sleep. It is therefore important to allow yourself enough time to let your body calm down and relax so it can tune in for a restful sleep.

Your body works at full speed all night; your organs do not take a break. Therefore, it is important to give your body the rest it needs so that it can go about its natural processes in peace and quiet and you can start your next day full of energy.

Following are a few examples of parts of an evening routine that you can incorporate into your life:
- Take a walk in nature.
- Meditate.

- Take a bath.
- Drink a cup tea or a delicious elixir (see chapter 7 for recipe ideas).
- Do yoga or some stretching.
- Read a book.

For your evening routine, it helps to set the mood by changing your surroundings. Light some candles, dim the lights, and snuggle up in warm comfortable clothes.

3.2 Food and mindset

Positive Mindset

The more you connect with your body and the more you pay attention to your body, the less you are in your mind or thinking mode.

This may sound very simple. But if you ask me, it's often easier said than done.

One thing I've learned over the past few years is that you don't have to feel good every day. It's normal to have bad days or bad moments. It makes a big difference to be mindful of those bad moments.

We can't change what happens to us, but we have control over how we react to it.

We tend to focus most on what we want and what we lack in our lives. Today, however, I want you to change your perspective. The more you focus on what you already have in your life, the more good things you attract into your life.

When you focus on what you have in your life, you begin to change your energy. And you always attract what we radiate.

Following is more detail about your mindset when it comes to food:

How You Think about Food Is Important

Eat food that brings you energy instead of taking it away.

Before you begin and move on to the following action steps, which I listed for you, take a moment for yourself to write in your journal what you really think about food. Do you love food? Do you enjoy food? Are you afraid of calories? Are you afraid of eating too much sweet stuff? What is your relationship to food?

Take time to answer these questions. Don't rush yourself.

When you're done writing, read over what you've written. Writing helps you go deeper. It's an amazing way to express what you otherwise keep hidden inside.

It allows you to dive deeper, possibly with things emerging that you never thought were there.

Since this section is about your attitude toward food, the first step to changing that attitude is to become more present. The more you are in the here and now, the more you will be aware of your hunger. Are you really hungry, or is that hunger connected to something else?

Perhaps you are craving that chocolate because you need love or a hug. Possibly you are craving something salty because of your stress level.

Action Steps:

1. Focus on Adding Something to Your Life, Not Cutting Something Out

If you ask me, this is a very important step.

You may have heard the saying "See the glass as half full and not half empty."

This action step is about doing this very thing. Starting today, you will see the glass half full and not half empty when it comes to eating.

Always look at it from the point of view of what you *can* eat, what is nutritious and good for your body. If you always focus on what you can't eat, or better yet what you shouldn't eat, then you will always look at the glass as half empty.

There are countless recipes that offer an alternative to foods that you might prefer to avoid or else enjoy in a balanced way so that you can provide your body with optimal energy.

See chapter 7 for recipes for foods that you can enjoy without a guilty conscience.

Balance Your Energy

We have already discussed the topic of male and female energy. This week we will consciously focus on these two types of energy.

Why is the balance of these two energies so important when it comes to nutrition?

An imbalance between feminine and masculine energy creates an imbalance in every area of life. And so it is with nutrition. Those who pay too much attention to calories or to the number of grams of fat, carbohydrates, or protein they eat place great emphasis on control. Diets are dominated by male energy. One adheres to a specific plan, a preset number of calories, or the portion size. In such a case, the body is prevented from being itself; it is always under control.

Too much feminine energy in eating causes one to let go of too much. You no longer have control over whether you eat one bar of chocolate or two. You let yourself go.

A balance between the two energies is very important.

You shouldn't weigh your portions or count calories. But you also shouldn't just let go. Take a few minutes to ask yourself where your focus is. Are you too controlling when it comes to food, or are you just the opposite? Have you been able to find your center and achieve balance?

As with the previous steps, writing helps you access your inner self and find the answers.

<u>Listen to Your Body</u>
What does your body want to eat today?

Have you ever asked yourself this question, or do you simply eat what you think you need to eat? Do you take enough time for your meals? Do you cook only what is in the refrigerator?

Take a few minutes to answer the foregoing questions. Write down the answers or feel them by paying attention to your body.

The next time you prepare a meal for yourself, ask your body, "What do you want to eat today?"

If an answer comes up such as "french fries," "chips," or "pizza," ask yourself, "Where did this answer come from?"

Often the body craves sweet, salty, or unhealthy things when, in fact, it needs something else, for example, affection or attention. Or maybe it's just stress.

<u>All about Balance</u>

It's what you eat most of the time that matters, not what you eat once in a while.

I personally live by the 80/20 rule, which means I spend 80 percent of my time making sure I'm fueling my body with healthy and nutrient-dense foods and the remaining 20 percent of the time enjoying whatever I feel like eating.

If you prohibit yourself from eating something, your body will want it even more. Forbid yourself nothing; enjoy in moderation. Practice balance with everything.

The most important thing is that when you indulge in a piece of chocolate or cake, ensure the proper sort of energy is behind it. As mentioned earlier, everything is energy. When you treat yourself to a piece of chocolate and eat it consciously and with pleasure, then the energy can flow; you don't block yourself. If you eat chocolate and feel bad afterward or even during, then the body takes this energy and blocks it, preventing it from flowing.

Allow yourself a piece of cake or chocolate. This is important, though: do it consciously and in moderation. Keep everything in balance:

To help transform your mindset to a positive one, ask yourself: "Where do I compare myself to others?"

Each of us is unique, which means we're different from everyone else. Everyone is on their own journey. Everyone has good and bad moments. Especially on social media, we see the perfect moments.

When you compare yourself to someone else, you are blocking yourself and your energy.

Always remind yourself that you are exactly where you are supposed to be. Every life is a book, and you are writing your own book. In every chapter of your book, you are exactly where you need to be. Don't compare your story and your book with other stories and other books. It's not the same book; it's a different story.

3.3 Cravings

Women often crave chocolate when about to begin menstruating.

Chocolate contains magnesium, which can relieve menstrual cramps. In addition, chocolate gives us a feeling of love. When we are looking for attention or love, we often crave chocolate or sweets.

When our body craves fatty and salty foods such as chips, the reason is that we're having stress. Fatty foods give us comfort in stressful situations.

When we feel a craving for something crunchy such as chips, it may be because we have suppressed anger that can be released by eating crunchy foods.

I remember when I read Kimberly Snyder's (celebrity nutritionist and holistic wellness expert) book called BEAUTY DETOX POWER, I learned for the first time how much our cravings are connected with our emotions. In this book, she describes in a much deeper way the connection of cravings and food.

The most important thing is to be present when a craving comes. Every time a craving comes, take on the role of observer. Ask yourself why you are having a craving for that particular food. You may get the answer right away, and it may be that you are simply stressed. Maybe it will take a little longer to notice why you have this specific craving. As I already mentioned, intuition needs to have practice in order to get stronger. The more you ask yourself, the more likely you'll be to realize why you are craving something specific. If you have a craving for something, it doesn't mean that you can never eat that food again. All that matters is that you enjoy it consciously and in moderation. How you eat something and the energy you bring t it is crucial. You need to bring the right energy so that your body can absorb the food and digest it completely.

As mentioned in the previous section, it is important that you acknowledge your feelings. It is important to truly feel how you feel, especially when it comes to food. Many times, we eat based on our feelings and not based on our level of hunger. The more you listen to your feelings, the more you will notice your cravings automatically disappearing. You won't overeat anymore as you will notice when your stomach is full and satisfied. The key is, when it comes to having cravings, to ask yourself why you crave that specific food.

When you ask yourself this question, you may want to sit in silence for a few minutes. You may want to take out your journal and write about your feelings. Practice one of the steps in *Nourish Yourself* to bring yourself back to the present moment and into the energy field of your body. By coming back to your body, you have the opportunity to dive deeper. You connect on a deeper level and have access to why you feel the way you do.

When it comes to cravings, I have learned a very important lesson.

Be Gentle with Yourself

There are many reasons why we might crave something. It could be based on our mood, our hormones, our feelings, a lack of nutrients, or actual hunger or thirst.

When I learned to just be gentle with myself, it was a total game-changer.

So today, I ask you to do the same: be gentle with yourself. Always tell yourself that you are doing your best, even if this is eating chocolate or cake.

Connecting to your feelings and listening to your body is an ongoing process. It takes practice to strengthen your intuition and to know what is best for you.

Remember, you are exactly where you need to be. You are only human.

Also, remember that some days you eat more greens and some days you eat more chocolate. It is about balance. Tomorrow is a new day where you can choose again. Don't be too hard on yourself. All I ask you to do is to be in the present moment. The more you connect to your body and the more you are in the present moment, the more you discover why you crave something. You learn the language of your body, also learning what is best for you and your body.

It is an ongoing process. It is a journey, so I ask you to take every step it takes you to proceed on your journey. Every journey is different as we are all unique.

3.4 **Masculine and feminine energy**

During my training to become an integrative nutrition health coach, I learned about feminine and masculine energy. I already knew about the yin and yang, or masculine and feminine energy. Given my interest in spirituality, yoga, and mindfulness in general, I have read a lot about masculine and feminine energy. To be honest with you, though, I had never consciously perceived them in my own daily life.

The turning point for me came when one day I realized how important it is to have these two energies in balance. I had been living and acting in an imbalanced way for many years and was totally unaware of it.

I was way too much in my masculine energy, which was dominant in every area of my life. When it came to sports, for example, I demanded far too much of my body. When it came to food, I controlled my intake far too much. I was exerting too much control over my portion sizes and was counting calories in my twenties, which behaviors are all about masculine energy. There was definitely no room for the feminine.

At work, I definitely didn't want to give up control at all.

When I learned how much easier and simpler it is to be and live more in my feminine energy, not only did lightness and balance come, but also everything was allowed to flow. I was finally living on allowance, allowing myself to be in a state where I could receive and where my body could recover.

Are you too much in your masculine energy? Are you perhaps too much in your feminine energy?

What can you do to balance your two energies, your yin, and yang, so that you can be more, receive more, and allow the energy to flow in your body?

Answer these questions calmly. Take your time, sit in a quiet place, and write down everything that comes to your mind after you ask yourself these questions. Just let it flow.

It is very important to feel the balance between these two energies. Also, I want to let you know that neither of these two energies is better than the other. It is important that you create a balance between both energies in your body.

There is a healthy masculine and a healthy feminine way to express feminine and masculine energy. It is important to express these energies in a healthy way rather than acting in a weak and unbalanced way.

Following are a few examples of traits arising from unbalanced male energy:
- dominance
- inability to be vulnerable
- being overly competitive
- being too focused on the outcome
- aggression.

Following are some examples of traits arising from unbalanced feminine energy:
- uncreativeness
- depression
- weakness
- having a victim mindset
- being stuck with regard to vision
- low self-esteem.

Following are a few examples of traits arising from balanced male energy:

- coming from a place of doing
- being giving
- mindfulness
- action
- specificity
- thoughtfulness
- being organized
- expressing oneself
- individuality
- being focused on results.

Following are some examples of traits arising from balanced female energy:

- allowance
- passion
- being emotional
- having vision
- flexibility
- being holistic
- softness
- focusing on feeling
- coming from a place of being
- stillness
- being intuitive.

Important: As I've already mentioned, neither of these two energies is better than the other. The most important thing is that you create a healthy balance between the two energies and act out of the healthy masculine and healthy feminine energy.

A person with balanced energy does the following things:
- Starts the day by being mindful, eating a nutritious breakfast, meditating, and doing some exercise.
- Takes inspired action.
- Focuses on his or her vision.
- Nourishes himself herself with high-vibration foods.
- Always takes time for self-care.
- Makes plans and implements them.
- Is well organized.

Exercise:

Take a closer look at healthy feminine energy and healthy masculine energy. Notice what unbalanced masculine and feminine energy looks like.

After that, ask yourself, "How is my balance when it comes to masculine and feminine energy?"

Are you acting too much out of masculine energy or feminine energy? Do you feel a balance in your life when it comes to your masculine and feminine energies?

If you do not see a balance in your life or if you notice that you do have a balance, but you are acting too much from the weak side of masculine and feminine energy, in what areas of your life can you make changes? How can you bring more of the healthy masculine and feminine energy into your life? How can you create more balance?

Finding a balance between these two energies is important if you wish to be more generally balanced in your daily life. I experience a balance between these two energies when I connect with my body and understand its needs.

As with every exercise, take small steps. It is important that you focus on your own pace. Don't get distracted. Take every step you need to take in order to better balance these two energies.

Embrace where you are and go from there. If you feel overwhelmed, take a step back and focus on your breath. Sometimes changing something in your daily life can be very overwhelming. For example, if you'd like to bring more feminine energy into your day and you find it hard to be creative, for example, tell yourself that it is okay. Embrace the fact that you are finding it hard to be creative. Embrace where you are and ask yourself what small steps you can take to change it. Perhaps there is a hobby you can begin to bring more creativity into your life. Maybe you can listen to your favorite song and try to sing it or dance to it. The size of the change you make or the step you take does not matter. Every small step you take is important. Change creates change. Once you start, you will see that it gets easier, and things start to flow naturally.

Wherever you are, whatever you struggle with, whether it is finding balance with your energies, creating a positive mindset when it comes to food, or finding more love for yourself, you are exactly where you need to be. I want you to trust the process. Start with baby steps and do these again and again. Take as much time as you need. Be gentle with yourself. Trust yourself and trust that you can do it. Start small, so that you create long-lasting changes for yourself and become the best version of yourself. Always focus on your path, go at your pace, and never forget that every step you take brings you closer to your goal and every change leads to more change.

4

Spirituality

We are spiritual beings in a human body. I firmly believe that there is a reason why we have come to this earth. We are all here to learn and to grow, each in our own way and each on our own journey. Yet we are all one. We are all energetically connected. Everything is energy. The chair I'm sitting in right now and the computer I'm using to write are nothing more than forms of solid energy. There is also subtle energy, for example, our feelings and emotions. The words I am writing here are also a form of vibration and energy. A few years ago, I read about an experiment about a mother who had bought three plants with her two daughters. One plant they named Positive; one they named Negative, and one had no name. Every day they said negative things to the plant named Negative, and they said wonderful, positive things to the plant named Positive. They paid no attention at all to the plant that had no name. The mother wrote in her book how the plants either wilted or blossomed properly. I have never done the experiment myself, but I am a firm believer that negative words leave us with negative energy and that positive words do just the opposite. Words leave energy in us, and our bodies unconsciously hold on to that energy. Therefore, I have emphasized many times in the foregoing chapters that it is important to allow the energy to flow in your body. It is important that your body does not unconsciously hold on to something.

Just as important as energy are our feelings. So, in the following section, I will go deeper into the topic of feelings. Why are the feelings behind something so important? Why do we so often think we need something, but in reality, it's just the feeling we're looking for?

4.1 **It's about the feeling behind things.**

It's about How Something or Someone Makes Us Feel

When we are looking for something specific, we are always compelled by the feeling behind it. For example, if we want to lose weight, then it is about how we want to feel in our bodies. We think that with a few kilograms less on our frames, we will feel accordingly. Do we want to have something else in our life, such as success, money, or recognition, or something simple such as more time for ourselves or a larger piece of the pie? If so, it's really about what's behind it. Again, it's about what that thing brings to us and triggers within us. Or rather, what we think we will feel when we have it. We spend many days, months, and even years wanting something we think we need. However, the truth is that we are looking for a feeling. We can get that feeling of recognition or even just a piece of the pie in other ways.

Therefore, it is important to recognize what feeling we are looking for. What is it that we want to feel in truth? Why exactly are we looking for this particular person or object? We think that only this object or this person can give us what we think we are looking for or need.

In my twenties and early thirties, I thought I had to have a career. I had an image that was firmly anchored in my head. My belief was that I would be worth more if I were successful. In truth, I was just looking for a sense of what I thought success would give me. When I started my own business, I thought that my work was only valuable when I reached many people and helped make their lives better. In truth, there was something completely different behind it, and it wasn't until I worked on myself more intensively that I realized what was actually behind it. It was not primarily success that I was looking for; it was something that was inside me all along. So often we look for the answer on the outside and get distracted. But the answer is always inside us. We are perfect just the way we are. Each of us has everything we need to be perfect; we just have to look inside ourselves for the answers to our questions.

I thought I needed success so that my work would become valuable. I thought I would be happier if I reached more people. The truth is, however, that I was merely looking for a particular feeling. When I realized that it was a feeling that I was in truth looking for, and once I found that feeling inside me, a great weight lifted from me.

Today, every time I catch myself thinking I need to be successful in order to be happy, I remind myself that the truth lies deeper. Today I know that I am looking for that feeling and that I don't get that feeling from success. I know that there are many wonderful things that I can do every day to make sure that I have and get exactly what I am looking for.

The question for you is, where do you think you need something to make yourself happier? Is it a change in your weight? Is it more success? Is it more money or maybe more friends?

With the action steps provided in this section, you'll get the tools to help you identify that feeling and the thing you're really looking for. You'll learn not only to identify what feeling you want to feel but also how to get it differently, without needing that thing you seem to think you need.

No matter what you may think you are missing in your life, the answer lies in a different place than you think.

Material things such as expensive clothes or creams give us a certain feeling that we try to create for ourselves. Therefore, it is often the case that a new sweater or a new dress gives us a lot of pleasure at the beginning, but after a few weeks, it often looks different. The feeling we are looking for is always hidden inside us. The secret is simply to find the connection to our inner self and to this feeling.

I discovered only a few weeks ago that I have spent too much energy on having more social contact in my life. I don't have very much close contact with people where I live. This led to the fact that every time I met someone I liked, I thought we were going to be friends. Each time I thought the universe had heard me and sent a wonderful friend into my life. I hadn't yet learned the lesson. The relationship never developed into the friendship I wanted until I realized that the truth, I was seeking was deeper than that: I was looking for a feeling. The universe *always* supports us. It may be very difficult at times to believe that. But every situation in our lives exists for us to grow and learn from.

When once again the friendship that I wanted didn't materialize, I asked the universe for the real reason. What was it that I had missed? The answer came quickly: I had completely lost my focus. I had wasted so much energy on bringing new contacts into my life that I became completely distracted on the outside. When I realized that everything, I was looking for was inside me, not only did I get back in my power, but also I felt lighter than ever. It had taken many years, but I finally learned the lesson. Today I know that I have many wonderful things in my life. The universe was just trying to steer me in the right direction. Today, whenever I feel that I need new contacts in my life, I focus on myself, my work, and my wonderful family. These things awaken a deep love within me that I can't describe. After a few seconds of putting my focus on something else, my whole being shifts, and I feel full of love and perfection.

You too will find this love and perfection within you. You will realize that you will not find it on the outside. You will not find it in food or in other people. It is there within you, and it will never go away.

Action Steps:

Take Time

Ask yourself, "Where do I think I need something to make me happier?" Is it a change in your weight? Is it a lack of success? Is it more money or maybe more friends?

Take time to answer these questions. Go to a place where you will be undisturbed and write the answers in your journal. Maybe you would like to light a candle or play some music in the background as you do this. Do whatever it takes for you to go into yourself, feel into yourself, and write what wants to emerge.

Find a Calm Place within and Feel It

Whatever you wrote down for the previous action step triggered a feeling within you. Sit comfortably on the floor or on a chair and let your body relax. Put your hands on your knees and breathe deeply. Now feel within what the words you have written down have triggered. Where do you feel these feelings in your body? Let the breath flow, keep your eyes closed, and allow what wants to come up to emerge. Do not repress anything; let the energy flow. Don't repress your feelings but let them come up so that they can flow out of your body.

Make a List of All the Things That Nourish You from Within

What makes you happy? It is important here to write down things you can do at any time, for example, go outside, take a walk, listen to music, or make yourself a cup of tea. What small things do you do in your everyday life that help you nourish yourself and make you happy? You'll see it doesn't always have to be taking a beach vacation or doing something else that might cost you a lot of time and money. The little things in your everyday life can give you just as much wonderful perfection. I love to read a book. Or whenever necessary, I plthe ay music that encourages me to dance. Find these little things for yourself and implement them whenever necessary.

Ground Yourself—Become Present

Too often we get lost in the stories we create for ourselves. I am the perfect example of this. I'll tell myself something and then I'll have just one negative thought, and the negativity just flows, causing me to lose myself completely. I lose focus on what is important: *to be present* and to be in my body.

Whenever you have moments like this, whenever you get lost in your own negative stories and emotions, take a deep breath and ground yourself. Come back into your body.

Ask yourself simply: "Where am I? Where is my body right now?" These questions will help bring your attention to your body.

Whenever we are away from our heads and come into our bodies with attention, we automatically find ourselves in the here and now. Everything else is illusion. We don't know what the future holds, and the past is gone, so it is important to let it go. All that matters is the now.

Therefore, whenever necessary, find your way into the now. Ask yourself where you are. Focus your attention on your body and feel your breath. Focus on your breath for as long as necessary. Feel how it flows in and out. Breathe in deeply, and with each exhalation feel yourself relaxing more and more. Feel how your body relaxes until it is completely relaxed.

4.2 Live in alignment with your body and the universe. Learn how to let everything flow.

In the previous section, we talked about the true feelings and reasons behind desiring something. The more you realize your intentions and feelings behind the things you desire, the more you live in your own presence, your body, and your power.

As with everything else, this takes practice. However, the more you go into yourself, listen to your body, pay more attention to it, and notice your feelings, the easier it becomes to understand not only your body's signals but also the lies your ego is trying to sell you. The ego has no access to silence. Therefore, it is important that whenever necessary, you take the time to go into yourself, connect with your body, and thus gain access to your true being.

In this section, I show you how you can start living in harmony with the universe and your body.

Unfortunately, it happens too often that we do not listen to the signals from our bodies or the universe. We are often too much on the outside and become distracted by externals. With the steps in this section, you will learn to be in tune with the universe and your body. Not only are you surrendering leadership to the universe, but also you are learning how to separate yourself from negative energy, feelings, and emotions. So often we hold on to negative energies, feelings, and emotions, which then take hold of our bodies. They manifest in the form of poor digestion, pain, a deep-seated fear in the body, or even excess kilos that build up like a protective layer in the body.

It is important that the energy in your body is able to flow freely. In order for you to have space for everything that life offers you, you need to detach yourself from whatever is holding you back from receiving it. Everything that prevents you from being and living your true self can be let go.

Action Steps to Live More in Alignment with Your Body:

Daily Mindful Movement

Movement is, in my opinion, the fastest way to change your energy. I'm talking about mindful movement, in particular, the kind of movement that takes you back into your body, away from your head and your thinking, and toward feeling.

The way you move your body, whether in a workout or just regular motion throughout your day, can make a big impact on how you go through your day.

The day I started with mindful movement was therefore a game changer for me. The mindful movement helped me to feel much more connected with my body, to be more mindful, and to live more in the present moment.

Feel Your Emotions

Many of us have been taught that we should suppress our feelings and emotions. I often find myself telling my children to behave properly, to be quiet, or if they are making a drama somewhere along the way, to stop. I try to be present in those moments and tell myself that it's important to let my kids externalize how they feel. If we always suppress our feelings, if we are unable to express them, then they become stuck in our bodies, preventing the energy from flowing freely.

I have read in the past, that ninety second is enough when it comes to letting our feelings flow freely. All it takes is ninety seconds, during which time we need to go within ourselves and truly allow ourselves to feel. Whatever wants to come up, whatever we feel, we allow it to flow out, so that it no longer sits inside us and later comes back to the surface in some other form.

Following is a simple and easy exercise that will help you to truly feel your emotions and feelings so that they can dissolve:

Exercise—Feel Your Emotions

For this exercise, sit comfortably on the floor or on your meditation cushion. You may even lie down if you'd like. By lying down on your yoga mat, your whole body can relax. I myself notice during meditation the tension I feel from sitting up. Sometimes it is easier for me to relax completely when I lie down. Therefore, I also like to practice meditation while lying down.

The important thing is that you relax, that you find peace, and that you are in a comfortable position.

Once you are ready, close your eyes and bring your attention to your breathing. Breathe in and out slowly, deeply, and firmly. With each breath, come more and more into your body. The more you come into the energy field of your body, the more your mind can calm down. The goal is to move your attention away from your head. Focus all your attention on your body.

What do you notice?

Stagnant emotions block the flow of energy in the body.

Where in your body are the emotions that you are not noticing or are not ready to notice? You may feel a lump in your throat or heaviness in your chest. It might also be that your hip or your back hurts. Pain may also be in your stomach area. Now let that pain or pressure come up. Gently place your hands on that part of your body. Feel as your hands bring light to that part of the body. Consciously give love and affection to this part of your body through your hands. Tell yourself and your body, your inner self, that it is okay, that everything is good and that it is protected.

Keep your hands on that part of your body for as long as you like.

Whenever you are ready, slowly release your hands and bring the focus back to your breath. Stay relaxed and feel the energy flowing through your body. Notice the love and security you have given yourself. Whenever you are ready, slowly open your eyes.

Maybe you want to write a few words in your journal. Perhaps something has come up that would like to put on paper. Maybe you'd prefer to just enjoy a moment of peace. Do whatever feels right. *Nourish Yourself* is designed to help you find your inner power and, in doing so, find peace and balance in your life. It's important to listen to your body and, especially after an exercise like this, feel what your body is asking for. Does it want more rest? Do you want to write down some words? Does your body need fluids? Try to feel your body and give it what it asks for.

You will see that it will become easier and easier to recognize the signals your body is sending and to give it what it asks for.

Let Go of Control

We cannot control what life has in store for us, but we can control how we respond to it.

We always have a choice. We can try to learn from any situation. We can question the reason for the situation, why it came into our lives, and what it wants to tell us—or we can let a situation completely overwhelm us. We are all human beings, and we all have moments when we get stuck when it seems that we can't go on or can't go uphill. However, we always have a choice. No matter how stuck you seem to be, how low down you think you are, you always have a choice.

I have noticed in the past that often what gives me the most support in moments like these is *letting go.*

How does it feel when you are allowed to just hand everything over to someone when you are allowed to let go and trust 100 percent that someone else will take care of you. In my darkest and lowest moments, I have learned to let go. This may seem easier said than done but it isn't. Trust in the universe, trust in your path, trust why you are here, and trust that you are exactly where you are meant to be.

The universe does not send you tasks that you cannot handle. Have trust in yourself. Trust also your way, the book that you're writing with your life here on earth. If you have trouble, just let go and trust. Try an affirmation or a meditation or try talking to your guardian angels or the universe. Whenever I get stuck, I direct my words to the universe. I feel that the moment I say my first word out loud, my energy changes, love, and security come into my body, I feel warmth, and I know everything will be all right.

Let me give you an example. A few days ago, I was planning to take my kids to storytime. We had a fifty-minute drive ahead of us, so we went to eat something beforehand. The place we wanted to go to was a bookstore that was celebrating its tenth anniversary and, for this reason, was holding a fairy-tale lesson for the little ones. Everything went great; my kids and I ate something delicious and were on our way to the bookstore with more than enough time. However, I hadn't considered that the whole mall was celebrating its ten-year anniversary. Also, it was raining, it was November, and people had nothing better to do than to go to this mall. It was pure chaos. There was no sign of a free parking space in the underground parking garage. My kids were getting really impatient, and time was flying by. I just couldn't find a parking space. I could already see us sadly turning around and driving fifty minutes back home without having attended story hour. But I did not let that happen. I could have given up and turned around and gone home. But instead, I spoke to the universe, asking what it would take for me to find a parking space, also asking for support and help. I asked what I could do to allow us could participate in the story hour.

Something magical happened. Shortly afterward, I spotted a couple running to their car. I quickly turned on my blinker as a sign that I wanted this parking space. A few minutes later, I parked our car in the lot. The kids and I arrived at story hour just a few minutes late. The kids loved it—had a wonderful time—and I was just thankful that I had handed over control and believed in something bigger than myself and that everything had come out okay.

This may be a small example, but I could write here of countless examples where I have passed control. Try it yourself. Start small. Where in your everyday life can you start to pass on control? See what happens. Likely you will see how much more fluid your life becomes when you start handing things over to the universe, your guardian angels, or a higher power that is right for you.

What Can You Learn from This Situation?

I am convinced that everything that happens to us happens for a reason, no matter how painful it may be at that particular moment. In the past, I was very happy to give myself up to the role of victim. Today I try to see every obstacle not only from the point of view of love but also as a possibility. I then like to ask, "What can I learn from the situation? What does the situation want to tell me?"

Whenever you encounter an obstacle in your life, whenever you are stuck, ask what the situation you are in wants to empty you of. While doing this, close your eyes and center yourself. Be complete with yourself when you ask the question. You may get an answer right away, or you may notice a change in your energy right away. It may also be that the answer takes a while to arrive. This is perfectly normal and not a bad thing. The answer may come completely unexpectedly at some point. I often get answers while standing in the kitchen. The important thing is that you are always open to receiving the answer so that it finds you.

Focus on What Is Working

Whenever negative emotions and thoughts take over, I focus my attention on what is going well.

What is going well in your life right now that you can focus on? Is it wonderful friends who love you and are there for you or your family? Are you having success in business? Or maybe things are not going so well in business but are going well in your personal life. Focus on the things that are going well in your life, which may be small things. Often when you start thinking about these little things, you start thinking about more and more things that are positive in your life right now. That's what happens to me almost every time. At first, it may seem difficult to think of something good when you are caught in a negative situation, but once you identify something positive, more things automatically follow. By shifting your perspective, focus, and attention to something new and positive, you change your vibration and energy. The universe rewards you with more positive things, and you see your mood improve automatically, along with your whole being and your energy.

Choose Love

Maybe this point may sound strange to you. Love is the highest form of energy. I have learned that whenever I look at a situation from the perspective of love, I immediately am back in my body and in the present moment. Whether it's in a conversation, in a negative situation, or someplace where I'm stuck, whenever I refocus and tell myself I choose to bring love to the situation it usually changes into something better.

Try this yourself. Choose to see a situation with love, and you will notice that your way of looking at it and therefore the situation itself will change. Too often our egos get in the way, preventing this from happening. Choose *love* instead.

Trust that you are being guided, trust the process you are in, believe in the big picture, and believe that everything is there for you to learn and grow from.

4.3 **The connection between food, spirituality, and self-love in terms of spirituality**

Nourish Yourself deliberately addresses the three topics of self-love, spirituality, and nutrition. I firmly believe that all three topics are very closely connected.

My own journey began with a change in diet. In changing the way, I ate, I found my way into self-love and spirituality. Of course, it doesn't have to be this way for everyone. However, you start on your path, and wherever that path starts, is just fine. Everyone on earth goes his or her own way. Everyone writes his or her own book.

I myself realized that from the moment I decided to change my diet and do something good for my body, especially for my digestion, my personal perception changed step by step. I started to notice which foods help my digestion and which ones make it worse. As a result, I became more mindful of my body. I listened when my digestion was not doing well. I used to bad-mouth my body once I was out of energy and suffering from bloating or something.

This changed. I started to look at the reasons behind it. I no longer resigned myself to my condition and was unhappy about it; instead, I was ready to change something. This commitment to myself led me to start thinking differently about myself. I became more understanding with myself. Automatically, my self-love changed as a result. I noticed that the more I listened to myself, the more I learned to speak the language of my body. This allowed me to feel more love for myself and my body and to love in a new and deep way. It was okay if I was having a bad day, if I had no energy, or if my digestion wasn't particularly optimal.

It wasn't just self-love that changed when I started listening more to my body and paying more attention to it. I also became more mindful, so I automatically got more and more interested in the topic of spirituality. I have always loved to read. One evening when I went for a drink with my neighbor, she told me about a spiritual teacher from the USA. I had never heard of the woman before, but what my neighbor told me made me curious. Back home, I googled the name and the book my friend had told me about. My neighbor had discovered the book a few months earlier by chance at a yoga retreat. I ordered the book and immediately read through it in one sitting. It is called *The Universe Has Your Back* by Gabby Bernstein.

As it happened to my neighbor, the book also set a stone rolling for me. I was not aware until then that spirituality is within all of us and always accompanies us. Small things such as loving your body, preparing a meal mindfully and with love, engaging in a mindful workout, or reading a book, or just allowing yourself five minutes of silence are all spiritual. I wasn't aware of this until then, and Gabby's book brought this point home for me.

No matter where your journey started or where you are today, one thing is certain: from the moment you decide to take care of your body and therefore yourself, you change your whole being.

I will talk more about how you can learn to choose and listen to your intuition in the following sections. Learn how to live your power, how to find your purpose on earth, how to become the best version of yourself, and how to live a life of abundance.

The moment you decide that you want to do something good for your body, be it through a change of diet, as was the case for me, or through another path, your energy, and your whole being change. No matter where your path starts or how you start on it, you will see that as soon as you start to do something good for your body and listen to it, your self-love will change. The spiritual side becomes more intense; you become more mindful and more present with yourself and your whole environment. When you start listening to your body, you learn to love it more and more. You learn what nourishes your body, especially what foods. Not everybody needs the same amount of food, and not everybody asks for the same foods. It's important that you give your body the things and the foods that it asks for. Don't question your own power. You alone know best what your body needs. Trust it.

In the following sections, you will learn how to strengthen this trust and how to understand the language of your body.

4.4 **Never give away your own power. Listen to your intuition.**

As mentioned in the previous section, it is important that you trust your inner strength. Trust that you know what is good for you.

I share with you in this section a few simple and, in my opinion, effective exercises that will hopefully help you find your intuition and listen to it in the future.

How Does Your Intuition Feel?

Do you remember moments in your life when your intuition showed up very clearly?

I invite you today to take yourself back to one of those moments. Take your journal and close your eyes for a moment. Recall a moment when your intuition showed itself clearly. Afterward, write down everything that comes to mind. It is important that you not get too deep into your head. Let the pen flow. Don't think that by connecting with this situation, this moment will show itself energetically again. Feel into it; that's what it's all about. The feeling that is inside you is what you should put on paper. Take your time with the exercise; write as long as you like.

Do you remember when and where your intuition first showed itself? Most of us do not even notice the moments when our intuition shows itself. Ask yourself when you felt deep inside that something was right but couldn't explain it.

After two weeks into my relationship with my current husband, then-boyfriend, I said to my parents, "I have found the one. This is him." My parents just laughed, but I knew it. I just felt it. I couldn't explain it. Of course, the relationship could have broken up after a few months. I had no guarantee that he would be the one. Today, almost fourteen years later, we are still together. We are now married and have two wonderful children. My intuition didn't disappoint me back then. Another moment when my intuition showed itself strongly was when I was pregnant with my twins. I also had a feeling with my first pregnancy, but with that pregnancy, the feeling was very different. I felt deep inside me that something was not right. I knew something was wrong. Still, the joy of being pregnant surpassed that feeling. After a few weeks, though, the reality caught up with me when the pregnancy ended.

The second time I got pregnant was with my twins. I will never forget the first visit to the doctor. It was not very pleasant. The doctor confirmed the pregnancy but, at the same time, told me that I should come back in a few days because it was very uncertain whether both embryos would survive. However, I knew that both of them would be fine and that I would give birth to both of them, and they would healthy. I can't explain it; I just felt that everything was going to be fine.

When in your life did you have a moment where deep down you felt you knew the right thing to do? Or maybe, like me, you had a feeling that everything was going to be okay. Intuitions such as these can show up in even in the smallest of everyday moments, for example, in daily decisions. You sense what is the right thing to do by choosing something else.

Our intuition is our daily companion. It is always with us and never lets us down. The problem is that often we don't really listen when it shows up.

After doing this writing exercise, you should have a sense of what your intuition feels like. Many of us go through our days not even noticing how often our intuition shows up. As mentioned before, it is always with us; it is our most faithful companion. It is up to us to notice it and listen to it.

If you are new to listening to your intuition, you may find it a bit more difficult in the beginning. Your intuition is like a muscle. The more you exercise this muscle, the stronger it becomes. If you hardly feel your intuition or don't really know what it feels like, that's not a problem. The more often you are willing to listen, the stronger it will show itself to you. As the saying goes, practice makes perfect.

Connect with Your Intuition

To help you become more aware of and listen to your intuition, I have another exercise for you. I personally do this exercise every day. It helps me not only to be more present but also to strengthen my intuition, so I notice and listen to my body.

In a quiet spot in your home, sit on the floor, on your yoga mat, on or your meditation cushion. You can also sit on a chair with your feet hips' width apart and firmly planted on the floor.

Focus your attention on your insides. Be aware of your breath. Breathe in and out at your own pace, feeling with each breath how your body slowly relaxes, and your breath slowly becomes calmer. Then close your eyes. Slowly place your hands on your belly. Feel deeply into your center, the center of your body. Continue to breathe deeply and calmly. Notice how you feel today. How does your body feel? Do not judge; just be the observer and keep breathing calmly. When you notice how you feel today, just feel the energy of it.

Then slowly draw your attention to your center. Feel your power, your inner strength. Enjoy the stillness, embrace the moment, and feel the space you create with this practice of stillness.

In the stillness you receive.

In stillness, your intuition is the loudest.

In this moment of silence, your intuition is strongest. You create space for your intuition to show itself. Feel clear how it is allowed to show itself. Imagine a situation in your life where your intuition showed itself. Feel how your energy changes when you imagine this situation with your eyes closed. Notice the moment when you clearly felt that your intuition was talking to you. Connect with this moment. Take as much time as you like.

Then slowly come back to your body, continuing to breathe deeply. When you are ready, slowly open your eyes.

Talk to Your Intuition

Another wonderful exercise to give your intuition space and strengthen it is to ask your intuition questions.

Connect with your intuition as described in the previous exercise. Again, take as much time as you like. Once you feel ready, ask your intuition your desired question.

If you are not yet as practiced at listening to your intuition, start with small questions. Maybe you ask it what good you can or may do for yourself. You can also start by asking what you should cook for yourself. Here you are asking not only your intuition but also your whole body what it needs, so you learn right away to listen to your body and give it the food it actually asks for. You can also just enjoy the silence while noticing what question is in the room. Sometimes you may not even be aware of what question is waiting deep inside you that would like to be answered. Feel deep within yourself, connect with your intuition, and let the question appear that is waiting to be answered.

Over time, you can let your questions become bigger. The more you talk to your intuition, the clearer its answers will be.

Remember that it takes time. Some people feel and recognize their intuition faster than others. Do not compare yourself with others. Your pace is the right one. Take all the time you need. Always remember, you are writing your own book. You are in your chapter, and this chapter is different from the other books and chapters.

Intuition and Nature

We are natural beings. Therefore, nature is a place of power for us. We can relax when we spend time in nature. We are connected to nature. The tranquility that nature gives us is not only the perfect place of power for us but also the perfect place to connect with our intuition.

Do you find it hard to connect with your intuition at home? Try taking a walk in the forest. The silence of the forest will help your intuition show itself. Feel free to do the previous two exercises in nature if you like.

It is a wonderful way to connect with your intuition by finding a quiet place in nature. Stand with both feet firmly on the ground. Feel yourself slowly becoming grounded and relaxing. Feel your breath flowing deeply in and out. When you are ready, gently close your eyes, place your hands on your belly, and feel your strength in your center. Feel deeply into yourself. Slowly, stillness and relaxation will flow through your body, and through this created space, your intuition will reveal itself. As mentioned in the previous two exercises, you can also ask questions about your intuition or can imagine a situation in your life where your intuition was allowed to show itself clearly. Again, take as much time as you need.

All three exercises can be done at any time. They are simple, yet they help you to feel and strengthen your intuition. The stronger your intuition is, the stronger your inner power becomes. You gain self-confidence and inner strength.

The more you do these exercises, and the more you give space to your intuition, the more it will show itself. However, it will not show up if you are not present. Intuition comes into play in quiet moments. Therefore, it is important that you give yourself space every day to connect with yourself, your intuition, and your body.

Over time you will learn and know exactly when intuition shows up by way of how it feels. As a result, you will question things less and less. You will know your way. You will feel from within what is right for you, including what is the right answer to a question and which is the right way for you. Your inner strength will become your most faithful companion. You can always rely on it.

4.5 We are all here for a special reason.

Follow Your Purpose and Step Out of Your Comfort Zone

We, humans, are creatures of habit, and we love being in our comfort zone. Breaking out of this cozy comfort zone requires energy and, above all, courage.

I am not asking you to change your life overnight. If you start to listen to your intuition, if you start to go through your day more mindfully, nourishing your body with fresh, healthy food and an extra portion of self-love, then you will automatically start to want to break out of your comfort zone.

By starting to listen to your intuition, you will automatically start to follow your purpose.

I firmly believe that we are all here on this earth for a reason. We are each a spiritual being living in a human body. We are here to have human experiences. We are here to learn and grow. The purpose of all our experiences here on earth is for us to learn and grow. That is why there is no such thing as an obstacle. Obstacles are like signposts; they either point us back to the right track or help us to learn from a situation.

Today I invite you to pick up your journal and take a few minutes to think about the following two questions:

- "What can I do today that will bring me a little closer to my purpose here on earth?"
- "What can I do today to break out of my beloved comfort zone, even if only a little bit?"

These questions are about being present, as with everything within these pages, to feel within and connect with your body. How often do you, like I sometimes do, go through the day, the weeks, or even the months forgetting your real purpose? Nowadays there is so much outside distraction that it is often difficult to keep the focus. These questions will help you to keep your real goal in mind. To follow your real goal here on earth, you must have courage and break out of your comfort zone. How many times have I wanted to stay in my own comfort zone so that I wouldn't have to stumble into the unknown. For the ego, the uncertainty is scary. The ego therefore often tells us that it is safer to stay in our comfort zone because we don't know what is waiting for us. However, this prevents us from living and realizing our true potential here on earth. It prevents us from pursuing our purpose on earth. We are all here on earth for a specific reason, and in order for us to live according to our true being, come into our power, and serve for the good of all, we must have courage and step out of our comfort zones.

The foregoing two questions will help you to take small steps. These small steps will bring you to your goal in the long run. You will become your true self and fully realize your potential on this earth. Let your light shine. Share it with the world. You are here to shine. All you have to do is follow your intuition, listen to your heart, and step into your power. That's why I'm writing *Nourish Yourself* so that you have support and a guide to help you do just that.

4.6 How to find your purpose.

As mentioned in the previous section, I am convinced that we are all here for a reason. We are here to realize our potential and to shine. We are all connected. The more light you bring to this earth, the more you invite those around you to do the same.

I remember booking a palm reading session many years ago. I was amazed at how much can be read in the palm of one hand. I found it very scary. The palm reader had said some things that were very scary to me. At the time, I was living happily in my comfort zone. I knew deep down that there was more waiting for me. But as I mentioned before, the unknown scares the ego, so I was afraid of it. The ego said that it was safer for me to stay in my comfort zone. Unfortunately, I listened to this voice of safety far too often, and, as a result, led a life that was not really meant for me.

We often forget that uncertainty brings many wonderful things along with it. That which is uncertain is not scary. That which is uncertain brings us magic and things we think about only in our dreams. The truth, however, is that anything is possible. We just have to firmly believe in it. We are infinite beings who have the power to draw magic into our lives. For this, we, need firm belief. We need to embody it 100 percent. We have to believe 100 percent that it is reality. If we live it and embody it 100 percent, we have the power to draw it into our reality. This is called manifestation. Maybe this sounds familiar to you.

The session with the palm reader taught me that I have to believe in myself. All the things he said, I felt deep inside myself. However, I never let them surface, being too busy living in my comfort zone. But that session, those things the palm reader said to me, made me think. I remember saying to him that I really only wanted this one thing. I wanted to play a small part in making this world a better place. I wanted it for my children, for myself, and for all the people who are here.

When I became aware of this and thought about these words over and over, I started asking myself the following question every morning: "How can I make this world a better place?"

At that time, I didn't know what my purpose here on earth was. Today I think my purpose is to listen to my heart, spread my light on earthe th, and follow my intuition. If you start asking yourself this question every morning, then every morning you are taking a step on your path. You are following your true path on the earth, the path that is meant for you, the path of your purpose.

As I write these lines and glance at the clock on my computer, I see that it is 11:11. I am firmly convinced that this is not a coincidence. The angels who write through me wanted me to give you this message.

Whether you know your purpose exactly or not does not matter. Follow your heart. Listen to the inner voice that guides you and shows you the way. Trust that you will be guided. Trust that every obstacle is there to put you on the right track, to put you back on your path. Every obstacle is there so that you can grow and can learn from it. Start to see these obstacles as something good. Remember and trust that you are writing your book and that you are exactly where you need to be. Trust your path to lead you. We are all on a journey, each of us on our own. We can't take over someone else's journey. We may cross someone else's path. We may walk a piece together. We may even walk together with certain people for a very long stretch. But there comes a point when people say goodbye again because they are destined to go another way. New people are allowed to show up on your journey. Be open on your journey. Be willing to learn, and always trust your heart, which will show you the way and guide you.

Now for some other considerations to help you determine your purpose and your path: If you had all the money in the world and time didn't matter, what would you like to do? What would you like to do if nothing and no one were to stop you? Of all the things in this world, if you could choose what you would like to do every day, what would it be?

Have you ever asked yourself these questions? If not, ask yourself the questions today. Pick up your journal, find a quiet place in your home, close your eyes, and take a few deep breaths. When you open your eyes again, read the three questions calmly. Take a moment and let the questions sink in. Perhaps you can already feel the energy around you begin to change.

If it helps you to answer the questions better, then retreat for a moment. You may want to enjoy meditation for a while so you can really get into yourself. Feel deeply into yourself. Connect with your inner self, your center. It's about getting away from your head. It is important that you answer these questions not with your thinking, but with your feeling.

As mentioned, many times in *Nourish Yourself,* we are all different. Here are two simple ways you can get answers to the questions without going into thinking mode:

1. Let It Flow

Sometimes it's a good idea just to write without thinking. Maybe this is just the way for you. Let the pen glide across the paper. Whatever wants to be on the paper, let it come up from your subconscious and write it down. Let your inner self, your intuition, take the lead. Let yourself be guided.

2. Meditate and Write in Your Journal

Enjoy a moment of silence. Take the time you need to let your body arrive. Ground yourself, sit comfortably on the floor or a chair, close your eyes, and breathe deeply in and out. Slowly bring your attention to your breath and to your body. Feel inside yourself and see what images come up when you consider the questions in front of you. You can also do a guided meditation if that is easier for you.

As with everything, there is no right or wrong way to find the answers. What is important is that you choose what is right for you.

Try not to fall into thinking mode. Stay in your body. Be aware of the energy. It will guide you and bring you to the answers.

It may be that the answers to these questions come as a complete surprise. It may also be that deep inside you have always known, or have known for a long time, what really brings joy to your heart.

Now that you've hopefully found some more clarity about what your heart is asking for, how can you bring more of it into your life?

In the following section, I share simple steps for inviting more of what your heart is asking for into your life, so you can follow your true purpose here on earth

4.7 **Become your best self and attract abundance into your life.**

We are each a soul in a human body. We have a task here on earth. We are all here for a reason. The problem is that we unlearn to follow our soul plan at a very early age. Instead of learning how to make our inner light shine, how to shine and share it with the world, we put it in the background. Things such as competition, career, material wealth, or social status take the forefront.

I hope that with *Nourish Yourself* you take the opportunity to find your inner light, feel your inner power, be able to live your true life and follow your heart.

It is important that you find your inner balance. Further on I talk more about feminine and masculine energy. I like to call it yin and yang. As already mentioned, this has nothing to do with your femininity or masculinity as a person; it is just about the energy. Both energies need to be balanced so that you yourself are in balance. Most of us have lost that balance, which is not surprising. If there is an imbalance on the outside, it is all the more difficult to bring yourself into balance on the inside. Everyday life is characterized by masculine energy, such as doing, being quick, competing, being controlling, and thinking.

Many of us also have the feeling that if we just do nothing for a while, if we just are, then we are lazy. I myself prevented myself from simply being for years. I had the belief that I needed to be productive. I had the belief that doing nothing meant I was lazy.

It wasn't until a few years ago that I learned how important it is to just *be* and get away from *doing*. I learned how important it is just to be in order to be productive. I've noticed that the more I allow myself to *pause*, the more productive I am. I've noticed that I only get in balance when I slow my pace every now and then.

How can I be there for others if I'm not there for myself?

How can I nurture others if I'm not nurturing myself?

Doing something good for others, wanting to help, is something wonderful. But ask yourself if you wouldn't make a far greater contribution to others if you were the best version of yourself.

How can you become the best version of yourself?

Have you ever asked yourself this question: "What is the best version of myself?"

Many of us are not even aware of the best version of ourselves.

What is your answer to that?

Honestly, I was never really aware that I actually had an answer to this question in my head, but my answer was different from reality. I unconsciously had an image in my mind created by external distraction. These days, the topic of wellness is omnipresent. Countless products are on the market. The goal of every company allegedly in support of wellness, of course, is to make us think we need their products. On top of that, spending time on social media has the effect of making us compare ourselves to others. We forget that what we see on social media is maybe 2 percent of the whole reality; we forget about the other 98 percent. On top of that, we may also fail to realize that the image we are looking at has been edited. We don't know the story behind it, or how it was created. We only see this small moment and the surroundings we create ourselves in our own thoughts.

As for myself, I had a clear idea of the best version of myself. I had an image in front of me of the person I aspired to be, a perfect person who had it all together had the perfect body, was successful, and was a wonderful mother and wife. As I mentioned before, the reality was different. It took time for me to realize that the best version of myself is a very different version. This person is far from the perfect image I was striving for. I was allowed to feel gratitude and love for my body. I started being kind to myself and my body. I started listening to my body. I didn't have to be perfect anymore. This realization changed everything. I didn't start letting myself go; on the contrary, I wanted to do good things for myself more than ever—me and my body. I started setting boundaries; I allowed myself to take more breaks, and I started nourishing my body with the best possible foods. With self-love, self-acceptance, and with foods that were good for my body and that it was asking for or demanding, I became the best version of myself.

What is your image of the best version of yourself?

To answer this question, you can use your journal to help you. Glide your pen across the paper. What comes up as an answer? Where do you have that particular image of yourself, the perfect version of yourself, that you may break away from today?

It's important to be clear about what image you have in your mind that you consider being the best version of yourself. To get clarity on this concept, you can just think about it, meditate, move into silence, or just let the pen flow. As suggested earlier, don't judge yourself for what or how you write. Let go of all expectations of yourself. There is no wrong or right. You are not good or bad at writing. The point of this kind of writing is to give you access to yourself to learn what's deep inside you, including any evaluations and also what power. What a wonderful person you are. It is time to show this to the outside world.

While this section is about being your best version of yourself, it's also about letting go of that perfect image in your head. It's about taking care of you and being willing to listen to your body and do good for it and for yourself. For example, give your body healthy nutritious food. Give yourself time each day for self-care. These little things make you the person you are, and the more you take care of yourself, the more you automatically become the best version of yourself. What small steps can you take in your everyday life to make yourself the person you've always wanted to be? It's not about becoming a model. No, it's about learning that you have everything you need. Give yourself attention and love to the little things in life and take care of yourself and your body. You have only one.

Let go more and more of "being perfect"; you are perfect the way you are. The only key is that you are willing to do good for yourself. Listen to your body, and nourish it with love, healthy food, self-care, and everything it asks for and needs. All it takes is for you to learn to listen to your body and pay attention to it. Detach from perfectionism and let your body relax. You will see, your whole being will automatically change, and you'll become the perfect version of yourself.

Always follow your heart and listen to it.

Maybe you expected something different when you saw the title of this section. From my own experience, through my work, I was able to learn that everything we think we need can be found within us. The answer that we so often are looking for on the outside is within us. So is the answer to inviting abundance into your life or becoming the best version of yourself. An important point, if you hope to find the answer to both these things, is to follow your heart. Start listening to your heart. Trust that your heart, and your intuition, will always show you the way. Mistakes are human and are important. Only from mistakes can we learn. By looking at mistakes not as mistakes, but as something we can learn from, we change the way we look at them, and so automatically our energy changes. The energy we emit is what we receive.

Do you want to receive more abundance in your life? If you start to listen to your heart, act out of love, and look at any mistakes you make not as mistakes but as a chance to learn something, then, as mentioned, you change your energy to positive and automatically attract more abundance into your life.

Bring Small Things into Your Life That Nourish Your Heart and Fill You Up

As mentioned, many times within these pages, everything is energy. With *Nourish Yourself*, I invite you to be more in your body, so that not only do you get more balance and strengthen your intuition, but also you automatically become the person you've always wanted to be. We all have our bad moments or even bad days. This is normal. It is important that you accept these moments and feel them so that the emotions are not pent up in your body but can flow away. However, it helps, especially in these difficult moments, to implement small things in your daily life that nourish your heart. As asked in chapter two, on self-love, what are small things in your life that nourish your heart? For me, it's spending time with my kids. I also love just dancing and listening to music or even taking a walk. When I do these little things, I automatically feel the energy inside me change. The smallest things can give so much nourishment and joy to your heart, which is transmitted to your whole being. The energy you radiate changes, as does the energy you receive.

Have a positive mindset, be willing to learn from mistakes, and see obstacles as opportunities.

I mentioned briefly in a previous point that obstacles and mistakes are important. They help us learn from a situation. You may already know that often we make the same mistake several times. There is a reason for that. We make the same mistakes several times so that we can see the lesson and learn from it. I try to ask myself with every mistake or obstacle in my life, "What does this situation want to show me? What does it want to teach me?"

When you ask yourself such powerful questions, don't expect an answer right away. However, trust that the answers will find you. Trust that the answers will come at the right moment. Another mantra that I have learned from different teachers over the years and always carry with me is "In stillness I receive." The answer to your question may arrive at any time, sometimes a few minutes after you ask the question. Sometimes it takes days. Stay confident that the answer will come. The answer usually comes very unexpectedly. However, it only comes when you are present. If you are distracted, then the answer has no chance to come to you. When you are in the moment, you are ready to receive what wants to come to you. Meditating can help. It can also help you to just be in the moment.

For example, I love to be creative in the kitchen. Very often when I am in the kitchen trying new recipes, I receive messages or answers. When I can be creative in the kitchen, it's like a kind of meditation for me. I am complete with myself, completely in my body, and that is the state where I and my body are ready to receive.

Of course, it doesn't mean that you must go into the kitchen either. Find a way for yourself to arrive in the moment. How can you be more in the now?

For many, it also helps to write down the questions. So once again, I invite you to take your journal and write down the questions. Maybe you will get the answer while you are writing. Maybe it will reach you later. Once again, trust that the answer will come. Trust that you can learn from the situation you asked about. Trust that you are not alone in finding all the answers.

When you begin to trust this, your body automatically relaxes. This means that it enters reception mode. Because only in relaxation is it receptive.

In conclusion to this point, I would like to mention *be gentle with yourself.* Take all the time in the world. Do not challenge anything. Don't be bad to yourself if something doesn't go as fast as you'd hoped. This also applies to everything else in your life and to all the other points in *Nourish Yourself.* Trust that you are in exactly the right place. You're going at your own pace, not someone else's. You are writing your own book. You can't skip a chapter.

Invite Love into Your Daily Life and Let It Guide You

Something I try to do every day is to be present with the energy with which I do things. We can't control what happens to us every day, but we do have control over how we react to it. We have the choice with what attitude we approach something. There are things in my work that I prefer to do and other things that I like to avoid. I assume it's the same for you. How do you bring more joy to the day when you do things you don't enjoy as much? Quite simply, by changing the way you look at those things.

A few years ago, I read a book by a German entrepreneur called Judith Williams. Judith was writing about her story—how it all started and how she came to be so successful. She worked hard to achieve her success. What fascinated me when about her story was the fact that she always put love into whatever she did. Even if she had to do a job at the beginning of her career that may not have been as glamorous as she wanted it to be, she always gave 100 percent, doing every job with love and heart.

I admit that I don't always manage to do that. I notice how I close up right away when something doesn't really interest me. My body contracts and my mind immediately go into overdrive or is otherwise distracted. Today I am aware of this. When I notice how I want to close up inside my body, I ask myself, "What might I learn here?" I try to go through my day open and eager to learn, and I invite you to do the same. Many of us have had enough of continuing to learn after school, college, or apprenticeship. But in my opinion, we'll never stop learning. I admit that may be a little more eager to learn than others. Nevertheless, I am firmly convinced that we have the chance to grow every day. I am convinced that we are here on earth to learn and grow. Our life is a wonderful human experience that we are allowed to have. It would be a shame if we did not take full advantage of it.

In what area of your life can you change your perspective? Where can you be more willing to learn and become an even better version of yourself? Where can you be more with your heart, not blocking yourself and, instead, letting yourself be guided?

4.8 **Back to basics.**

Something I have learned over the last few years is now one of my daily mantras: "Back to basics."

Not only is this mantra my daily companion when eating, but also it has become one of my favorites.

We live in a society that presents so much outside distraction. Everywhere we turn, we find advertisements for products being touted to us that we are supposed to think we need.

Do you know that feeling after you clean out your closet, for example, the feeling when you bring order to a part of your life and dispose of old things?

So often we feel as if we need a lot of things to be happy. Yet the truth is often just the opposite. I am writing these lines at the end of the year. At this time, I often go into myself, retreating a bit, so I can reflect on the year. I think about what the year has taught me, what my wins and losses were, and what I want to invite into my life in the New Year.

Today I invite you to do something similar. Today is not about reviewing the old year, but more about inviting more peace and balance into your life.

I invite you today to invite less into your life. Where in your life can you cut something that will give you more ease and peace afterward?

We can't dance at all the weddings. If we do, then sooner or later we lose our balance.

To make sure you don't lose your balance, feel free to get out your journal and write a few thoughts about your life and your daily routine. Where can you invite more peace? What can you do or delete so that calmness finds its place?

Maybe you are someone who likes to say yes to everyone around you, so you are always cooking up new things to take care of.

Maybe, like me, you just like to take care of others and, in so doing, get out of your own way. There are always new people coming who need your help, even if they don't primarily ask for it.

Take the time you need and answer the following questions in your journal:
- "What can I eliminate from my life to make more room for calm?"
- "Where in my life can I invite more rest?"

Remember, less is more. And so, it is in daily life. Less brings you more balance, serenity, and calm. You'll also realize that when you accept less, it doesn't mean you should do nothing. By creating more balance and calm for yourself, not only will you be able to think more clearly, but also you will be productive and efficient.

How much do you like to get bogged down in chaos? By being calm, this doesn't happen in the first place, so you always stay on top of things, staying efficient and productive. You are operating from a different energy field, an unstressed body, and that transfers to your actions and deeds.

You can always come back to these questions. Everyday life is fast-paced, and it changes. I myself come back to these questions frequently. I take the time whenever necessary, and I invite you to do the same.

4.9 Surrender to the flow of life—let go.

I could possibly write half a book on the topic of surrender, which has been with me for several years and the past two years intensively.

Maybe you are like me, and you mark places in the books you read. Perhaps you include a note in the margin. Although I do this with almost every book I read, I put the book away after I'm done and rarely, if ever, pick it up again. There are a few books that I read more than once. Most of the time, however, I read a book only once. If it is the same for you, then I hope the message of *Nourish Yourself* has reached you. I hope that you will connect more with your body, follow your heart, bring your power to bear in the outside world, listen to your intuition, and share your light with the world. Every single line of *Nourish Yourself* is meant to help you to arrive at yourself, love yourself, accept yourself, and be grateful for yourself. Every line of *Nourish Yourself* should give you motivation and support to trust yourself, believe in yourself, come into your balance, and share with the world your power, your light, and the love that you carry within.

Another message I would like to pass on to you today is this: surrender to the flow of life.

I have written about trust again and again in *Nourish Yourself.* I want you to learn to trust yourself and your path here on earth. Remember, obstacles and mistakes are good things. They are there so that you can learn from them and stay on your path.

The important thing is not to get distracted by outside things. Whenever you get lost in a situation, think back to the exercises within these pages. They are simple and can be done anywhere and at any time. Maybe you put *Nourish Yourself* on your nightstand as a reminder, and whenever you need a little support, you go back to one of the exercises. At some point, these little exercises will become an integral part of your daily routine, and you'll notice how nothing can upset you so easily anymore. However, if there are moments that upset you, that's perfectly fine. You are still human, and as mentioned, you are here to learn.

Trust yourself and trust that all that is meant to be, will be.

I could list some of these things. The same goes for people who have suddenly come into my life. This year alone I have met many new and wonderful people. Some relationships were very intense and brief; others were with people who are still in my life. I am excited to see what journey I get to walk or share with them.

When I was little, I loved to write diaries and letters. I loved to read even as a little girl. In my teens, I slowly discovered a love for fashion, which became more intense in my twenties. I dreamed for years of being a fashion designer or fashion stylist. Another dream of mine was to work for a fashion magazine, be it as a stylist or even a writer.

Food and I were not friends until my thirties. On the contrary, I suffered a great deal from irritable bowel syndrome in my twenties. I had severe digestive problems. I was also ashamed of it and tried many things to improve my digestion—unfortunately, all in vain.

It was never my intention to gain a foothold in the field of nutrition. Before my children came into the world, I hardly spent any time in the kitchen, has always said that I would marry a chef so that I would never have to cook myself and have him prepare delicious food for me. I did not marry a cook, but my husband has a great passion for cooking, and so it was he who wielded the wooden spoon for the first seven years.

An interest in food and cooking came gradually to me. Out of nowhere, I started reading food blogs. I started spending money on cookbooks and tried my hand at cooking. A few months after my kids were born, I decided to change my diet. I didn't want to follow a trend; I just felt something inside me. I wanted to change for me. As I mentioned before, I suffered a lot with my digestion, and it also turned out that my hormones were not in balance. Therefore, I did not have an easy time becoming pregnant. On the contrary, the road was rocky, taking me longer than it takes many others. Today I look back and am grateful for this time. It taught me many things. And, as I said before, obstacles are here to learn from.

The decision to change my diet crept up on me little by little. Looking back today, I can't explain in detail why I made it at the exact time I did. I just felt it. I made the decision to change just a few things about my diet. I had no idea where this step would lead me or that it would turn my whole life around.

As I mentioned earlier, it was not my intention to work in the nutrition field at the time. The change in my diet resulted in a tremendous improvement in my digestion. In addition, after a few months, my hormone levels were back to normal, and I had a regular cycle. I was amazed at the effect nutrition could have and wanted to share news of this. I started holding small workshops and telling participants about it. I wanted to pass on how important it is to eat fresh, unprocessed foods. Also, I cut out industrial sugar by 80–90 percent. I have never forbidden myself anything, which is why I write "80–90 percent" here. Because I live according to the motto "Everything in balance." If I wish to have one piece of cake or one scoop of ice cream, then I allow myself. The more we forbid ourselves something, the more our bodies demand it, so I don't forbid myself anything.

The journey went on and on. I wanted to learn more about nutrition, so I enrolled in online courses. Wanting to share this knowledge, I created my first website with the help of my husband and started writing blog posts and creating recipes to share with my readers. More and more people came to me asking for recipes. In addition, they also said, "Why don't you start your own business?" However, I wasn't that far along at the time. The thought was rather scary.

Over the years, my interest in nutrition, exercise, and wellness in general grew. My passion, which used to be fashion (don't get me wrong, I still love fashion today. I love my clothes. I love dressing nicely, reading fashion magazines and blogs, and educating myself about fashion), transitioned into a passion for nutrition and wellness in general.

Never in my life would I have thought this would happen. I was embarking on a new path that I never thought I would take. I wasn't resistant to these things either. I felt inside that I wanted to change my diet. I didn't have an answer for it; I just did it. I started doing workshops. My interest in nutrition was increasing. Because I was feeling so much better, I wanted to know more and share my knowledge. It was a creeping process. Looking back today, I see that this is one of many examples in my life where I just went with the flow. Putting up no resistance, I let myself be led. It was destiny. I surrendered to the flow of life.

I want to pass on to you today that you, too, may surrender to the flow of life. Just letting go is very scary. It means to let go of control. Letting go of control means making room for the unknown. Anything we don't know is usually associated with fear. This is also the reason we like to get comfortable in our so-called comfort zone. It gives us security. Anything we can control gives us stability and a sense of security. But it also means that we will never live up to our potential. By succumbing to this sense of security, we automatically make ourselves small.

But what if you know that someone is taking care of you? What if you trust that the universe, God, or whatever you want to call it is with you and guiding you?

It may be very scary just to let go and be guided. I never really could do either. However, one day a book found its way to me, *The Surrender Experiment* by Michael Singer. Michael describes his own journey in this book, including how he decided to surrender to the energy of the universe. He has surrendered to the flow of everyday life. This book taught me that while I may think I know what is best for me, the truth is something else.

When I started listening to my heart, it took me on a new path. This path will never end. Not for any of us. One-stop on my path is to write *Nourish Yourself,* which I am writing for one reason: Deep in my heart, I feel that it needs to be written. It is something that I cannot explain. I feel it inside me.

I have been convinced for as long as I can remember that we are all here for a reason. When we learn to surrender to the flow of life, the real reason we are here on earth is allowed to reveal itself.

When you too surrender to your flow of life, you automatically release yourself from resistance. You no longer block yourself, so you begin to receive guidance, the guidance you need to go your way. You will be shown in different ways which steps you have to take. And never forget obstacles are there to learn from.

It is not easy to let go. Start with small things in your life. Where in your life can you start to let go? Maybe with your children? The older they get, the more they stand on their own two feet. As a mother, I know how difficult it is to let these little people go. Even though my children are still relatively small, it's already difficult for me.

Maybe you can let go of control at certain steps and hand over that control to someone else? Maybe you can let go of the need for perfectionism?

Try your hand at letting go in small ways.

Believe me, I have days when the control gets the better of me and I have a very hard time letting go. As they say, practice makes perfect. Don't be too hard on yourself. Give yourself all the time in the world.

Ask yourself the following question about letting go: "How does it feel to know that I am being guided and that everything that is meant for me will come to pass?"

Write the answer in your journal. Feel it.

It is not enough simply to look for an answer. Every exercise in *Nourish Yourself* is about feeling the answer. Feel it with your body. Feel the energy. Notice the energy that permeates your body and write down whatever comes up.

The whole of *Nourish Yourself* is a guide to teach you how to feel, be in your body, and receive.

Following is a meditation exercise to help you release:

Meditation—Surrender

This meditation is one of my favorites. I practice it several times a week. It helps me to let go and vibrate in the energy of the universe and thus be in the flow of life. Moreover, this meditation gives me confidence, support, and lightness at the same time.

I hope it will also help you to let go more and more and find the lightness and flow of your life.

You can practice the meditation lying down or sitting up. I myself choose the position depending on how I feel that day.

The important thing is that you relax, let go, and allow yourself to find the flow of life. Meditation is about incrementally letting go of the fear in your body, the fear that keeps you from embodying your true potential on earth, the fear that blocks you and makes you small. With this meditation, you will be allowed to release yourself from this fear and find the flow of life.

Find the position that is right for you. Sit comfortably on your meditation cushion, floor, or yoga mat, or lie comfortably on a mat on the floor. Slowly close your eyes and bring your attention to your breath. Notice how it feels as you inhale and then gently and calmly exhale. Breathe in and out at your own pace, calmly and gently. More and more you will connect with the silence. Embrace the silence. Whenever thoughts arise, let them gently pass by like little clouds.

Slowly feel how the heaviness disappears. Notice where in your body the heaviness is that is allowed to slowly disappear. Where is this heaviness in your body that manifests into fear? Let it go. With each exhalation, feel how you free yourself more and more and become light as a feather.

Imagine that you are as light as a feather. Feel how your body takes on the weight of a feather. The lightness carries your body, and it floats as gently and lightly as a feather.

Feel how your body becomes a feather that embodies pure lightness. Notice how white light appears around your body. This light carries you. Your whole body is enveloped in this white light that carries it. Notice how you become one with the flow of life. Your body and the light are one. They are connected. Your body is in tune with the flow of life. It floats and is carried and guided. You do not have to do anything. You may only be and let yourself be carried by the lightness.

Whenever a heaviness should appear that wants to pull you down, feel how the light helps you to ascend higher and higher. The light is stronger; it carries you, whatever comes. It holds you; it does not let you go. Trust that you will be guided by the light, the flow of life.

Let yourself be carried by this light as long as you want. It is with you. It never leaves. It holds you. Take this light with you as your daily companion.

Whenever you are ready, slowly come back into your body. Be aware of your breath. Breathe in and out gently and slowly a few more times, then slowly open your eyes.

We are all connected to this light, the flow of the universe. It is within us, entwining our bodies. When we allow it, we feel it. When we are in the now, it has access to us. Also, during the day, try to connect again and again with your light, the flow of life. Perceive it and feel it.

The more you allow it, and the more you strengthen your connection to it, the more you will see that you are ready to be in tune with your flow of life. You will realize that everything becomes easier. Doors will suddenly open that you never dreamed would open. People will come into your life. Things will happen out of the blue. Because you are in the flow, the universe may show you the way. And it leads you.

Trust in it!

5

Your Daily Guide and Daily Support

Whether your journey has just begun, or you are already far along the way, be assured that it will never stop. Life is there to grow. I subscribe to an app on my iPhone, the *Spirit Junkie* by Gabby Bernstein. Every morning it shows a new affirmation for the day. Today's affirmation couldn't be more appropriate for this chapter: "I show up for this life with a desire to learn and grow."

Every situation in your life, everything that happens to you, is there to grow from. In *Nourish Yourself* you have now been given some tools you can use so you don't lose focus. These tools help you to ground yourself, stay with yourself, and to grow. The exercises are your daily companion. We all have moments when we lose focus, when we are not in our center, and when we lose ourselves completely to outside demands. Whether you have just started or are far along does not matter much. What matters is that you always try to do your best, listen to your inner self and your power, and connect with it so that it can grow like a muscle. You will see, it will become easier and easier for you. Practice makes perfect. Be worth it. Put yourself first. Work on yourself and your growth so that you embody and live the best version of yourself.

You have seen in *Nourish Yourself* how important the right energy is for your body. Whether it is in the form of self-talk or in the form of food, it's important to let the energy flow, to not hold on to anything. Whenever necessary, let go. Trust that you are being guided and that there is someone higher watching over you.

I have written a small summary for you. Regard it as your companion and your support whenever you need it.

Keep *Nourish Yourself* handy on your nightstand or office desk. At the right moments, turn to the necessary page to support you in being grounded, finding love, or providing whatever support you need at that particular moment. If you do desire, let the book be your guide, your companion, and your support.

Summary

I wrote *Nourish Yourself* based on everything I learned during my journey. Every step represents a part of my life. Like everyone else, I have moments when I feel overwhelmed and when I look for guidance and support. It's important not to push those moments away. I used to run away from them. I always suppressed my true feelings, my true being. With my star sign, Cancer, I am very sensitive and close to the water. This was often rubbed in my face, and I always thought it was a bad thing. Today I know that this is a part of me. I don't have to hide or be ashamed of it anymore. Today I am proud of all my positive and negative qualities. Because the truth is this: We all have positive and negative qualities. It is important that we acknowledge them and embrace them. There are always two sides, yin and yang, plus and minus, or black and white. The balance is what makes the difference, along with how we deal with our negative and our positive qualities. It is the same with the dark and light moments in life. There are always both.

I once read, "Embrace the ebbs just like flows."

I don't think it could be put any better. Without bad moments, the good moments cannot arise. It is often the case that after the darkest moment in life, the light shines brighter than ever.

Whenever you have less productive days, whenever you have bad moments in your life, embrace them. Don't repress your feelings. These moments are important. They are there to show you something. Let them come up. Feel those moments so that they are allowed to move away again.

Of course, there are phases in life when you might like to let yourself go. That is completely okay. However, it's also important that you don't completely stray from our path.

I too have these days. From a nutritional perspective, it could be described like this: Some days are more about greens, and some days are more about chocolate.

However, it helps when I ask myself the following question:

How Bad Do I Want to Feel Good?

It is a question of setting priorities. Ask yourself the question when you go off course. How bad do you want to feel good?

Maybe you'd like to answer this question in your journal. You may feel the answer directly when you ask yourself the question. How can you set your priorities now so that they support you in getting back on your path? Can you perhaps start your day with a healthy, delicious breakfast that gives you energy and helps you be focused, nourishing your body and giving it what it needs to perform at its best? Can you schedule more time for your daily self-care regimen? Maybe it would help to do a little meditation, take a walk in the woods, or take a bath? Or maybe you want to move your body more and start with yoga or Pilates?

Remember, it takes only small things in your daily routine to support you in getting and staying on track. Go at your own pace. If you can't make it happen, find time for yoga or Pilates. Maybe start with five minutes of stretching and take the stairs more often. Where and how can you start? Small changes automatically lead to big changes. One change in your life automatically leads to the next.

Never forget you are exactly where you need to be, right here, right now.

Celebrate Your Wins

Something I learned some time ago that helps me to stay on my path is to celebrate my wins.

It doesn't matter how big or small these wins are. In fact, it's important that you celebrate even the small wins. My kids and I tell each other about every night at dinner what we are thankful for. Further, we tell each other what we thought was the greatest thing about the day. We review the day that way. We look at everything that happened to us and celebrate our wins that way.

Maybe you have heard about practicing gratitude. I will write more about practicing gratitude later in this section. Practicing gratitude and celebrating wins helps you to focus on the positive in your life. Gratitude is one of the highest and most beautiful forms of energy. Those who are grateful feel love, and love is the highest form of energy.

How often do you experience moments or even days when nothing seems to work? It is easy to get completely lost in these moments and see the negative. When you start celebrating your wins every day, though, you are much less likely to get lost in those bad moments. Your focus and perspective change by focusing on your wins.

Whatever happened during the day, there is bound to be a winner among those events that you can celebrate. However small or large that win may be, size does not matter. What matters is the fact that this win exists. Take a short moment in the evening to review the day. If you'd like, write down your wins in your journal. What happened to you today that you can celebrate?

As mentioned before, it may be a big thing, such as landing a new client or an important contract. However, it can also be a small thing, such as a smile from a stranger or the fact that you drank one less cup of coffee than usual.

On certain days, you may have a hard time finding wins. Believe me, they are there. You just have to look harder. It may turn out that things you thought where losses are actually wins. In addition, you may notice as soon as you write down your first win, that the second one is right behind it. Suddenly, you'll think of more and more things to celebrate, and you'll realize that the day wasn't as bad as you originally thought it was.

The purpose of celebrating your wins is to change your perspective. We tend to overlook the positive and focus on what is not going well. With this little exercise, you'll do exactly the opposite. You'll focus on everything that is going well. Most importantly, you'll learn to see the little things. Isn't it true that there is often great magic in these little things? Or is it the little things that count? Often the smallest things bring us the greatest joy. My children are the best example. It's those little moments with my children that make my day wonderful and precious. It's that laugh from my kids when they see me when they get school out and I'm waiting for them, or that deep gratitude I see in their eyes when I give them my attention when they're dying to show me something.

Sometimes, no matter how deeply you search and look, you still find it hard to discover a win. There are those days. Embrace them. Don't try to force a win or bathe yourself in your self-pity. Accept the moment, accept the day, and try to see each win as a gift from heaven.

It is such days that lead us to bright and shining days. Without darkness, there is no light. Remember, everything is here for you to learn and grow. And maybe the wins on such days are hidden or show up at first rather as losses—but when you look closer, they transform into wins.

It is always a question of perspective, and therefore it is always worth a second look.

A win can also be a shed tear, the sign that you have freed yourself from something and let go. A tear can also be a sign of something new that is waiting for you.

It's always a matter of your perspective!

Celebrate your wins. Celebrate every little step in the right direction. This will help you attract more of what you desire into your life. The more positive energy you radiate, the more you receive.

Celebrate yourself, celebrate life, and celebrate your daily wins.

Practice Gratitude

Just as important as celebrating your daily wins is practicing gratitude. I don't mean that you sit down every morning and write a gratitude list. I want you to feel gratitude. Gratitude is nothing but a form of energy. I want you to learn not to just write this energy on a piece of paper, but also to feel this energy with every fiber of your body. Learn what gratitude feels like.

This applies to everything in *Nourish Yourself.* I don't want you to do the exercises I share herein without feeling them. It's all well and good if you follow the exercises within these pages. However, the most important thing is that *you feel it!*

Maybe you've heard of the gratitude list. Wonderful. There is absolutely nothing wrong with making such a list. If you're already writing down what you're grateful for on a daily basis, then please, keep writing your gratitude list.

However, starting today, I want you not only to write the list but also to feel gratitude.

If you haven't started writing down what things you are grateful for in your life, I invite you to start today.

The Gratitude List

Every day, write down at least ten things that you are grateful for. It may sound like a lot, but believe me, once you find one item, more items will follow. You will change your perspective as with celebrating wins by focusing on the good in your life.

What are you grateful for today?

It doesn't matter how big or small the thing is that you are grateful for. It can be the running water that comes out of your faucet, the warm water while you shower, or the smell of the coffee you drink in the morning.

As you write your gratitude list, keep one very important thing in mind. Unfortunately, this part often gets lost. It is wonderful that you are writing your gratitude list, but don't forget to feel what you are writing. As mentioned, many times in *Nourish Yourself*, everything is energy. When you write your gratitude list, it's not about finding as many things as you can to be grateful for; it's about getting into the energy of gratitude. The real goal of the gratitude list is to come into the energy of gratitude and to operate from this energy. The easiest way, in my opinion, to get into the energy of gratitude is to write down what you are grateful for.

For example, if you are grateful that the sun was out today, consider how it felt, how the warm rays felt on your skin. Or if you wrote about being grateful that you spent time with your children, remember how it felt when you were playing with them. I close my eyes and take a moment to feel the things I am grateful for. After writing your gratitude list, you should also take time to meditate so that you can really feel and absorb the gratitude.

As mentioned, many times before, there is no right or wrong way. The way that is right for you is the one that helps you feel the energy of gratitude.

Morning Routine

I have written already before about the importance of having a morning routine. However, as this section is a little summary for you, I would like to pick it up again. I can't emphasize enough the importance of having a mindful morning routine.

Having a positive and mindful morning routine sets the tone for your whole day. Create a morning routine that you look forward to doing every day.

I can't emphasize enough how important your morning routine is. Since I have implemented a morning routine myself, my whole life has changed. Each night I look forward to the next day's morning routine. Thanks to my morning routine, I feel grounded and centered. I am more in my power, and as a result, I automatically go through my day more productive, more present, less stressed, and in balance. Time and time again I read from successful people that their secret is having a morning routine.

Would you like to have support in your life? If so, then create a morning routine. You can simply go back to section 2.8 and learn again how you can build your own morning routine which is right for you.

It's important that you find a morning routine that works for you. Every night before you go to bed, consider what you look forward to for the next day. What nourishes you? What helps you to get into your power and into your balance and, thus, to get through the day grounded and stress-free?

It took me months to find the right morning routine for me. I have to admit that I often looked outside myself to see what morning routines others had. In the beginning, I always tried to copy someone else's morning routine, thinking that it would have the same effect on me as it had on them. Sometime later, I finally realized that I had to look for the answer in myself. I needed to find out which morning routine was right for me.

And that's what I want to pass on to you, and not just with regard to the morning routine. Find the solution within yourself. Don't look outside; look inside yourself for the answer. I hope that with the help of the exercises within these pages, you will learn to communicate more and more with your body, listen to it, and speak its language.

So which morning routine is right for you and your body?

Of course, there are suggestions in chapter 2 that you can implement. Starting the day mindfully and with self-care is, in my opinion, a must when it comes to the perfect morning routine. But what kind of meditation and how long you should meditate is what you must find out for yourself. Do you want to do a guided meditation, do a breathing exercise, do mantra meditation, or just enjoy the silence for a moment? The point here is that you find what is right for you.

How do you want to move your body in the morning? Is a short stretch enough for you, or do you require a powerful workout?

A friend of mine once told me that putting on makeup every day was a kind of meditation for her. She is one with herself, is complete with herself in the here and now when she puts on makeup and gets ready. I myself feel this way when I am baking or creating new recipes. For others, that would be stressful and not peaceful. Where do you find peace? Where are you at one with yourself?

Take the time you need to develop your perfect morning routine. The important thing is to start the day being mindful and present. As mentioned, your morning routine sets the tone for the rest of your day.

Our morning routine is often the only period of the day we can control. We decide how we get up and how we start the day. Often, we can't control how the rest of the day goes. There are unexpected emails or meetings that don't go as anticipated. Maybe the kids are sick, or we are stuck in traffic. Very often we are not in control of what happens to us during the day. However, we are 100 percent in control of when and how we start the day. This start gives us the basis for the rest of the day. It gives us support and helps us keep a clear head in stressful situations. The morning routine is our support, is our rock, and helps us to be in our power.

Stop comparing yourself to others

I used to compare myself to others every single day. I was very good at comparing myself with others. I remember my high school days very well. At that time, I didn't realize how unique we all are. All I wanted then was to belong. I spent my high school years pretending a lot just in order to belong. Those were not easy years for me. I had made a few friends, but on the inside, I felt empty and misunderstood. I thought there was something wrong with me, and I was always comparing myself to the other girls in my class. I didn't understand why I couldn't just be like them. That didn't change later either. I didn't feel like I belonged for years. I kept wondering why I couldn't just be like other people, always thinking there was something wrong with me. As a result, I never really dared to be myself. I am very grateful that I was allowed to learn, and today I know that I am just right the way I am, that there is nothing wrong with me. Each of us is just right the way we are. We are all unique. We all came into the world with our own fingerprints. This fingerprint will not exist a second time. We all have light inside us that is ready to shine.

Carry your light out into the world. Never forget that you are unique. You are here to write your own book, and with each chapter, you are exactly where you need to be. Trust that you are guided. Trust your process. Trust the bigger picture of your life. Don't look to the left or right. Go your own way at your own pace that is perfect for you.

Embrace the ebbs as much as you embrace the flows of your life.

This sentence has changed my life. I heard it some time ago from Bondi Guru (bondiguru.com). In Bondi Guru's wonderful intuitive horoscopes, she mentions this phrase a time or two. It took me a while to learn to embody the phrase.

Our lives are full of ebbs and flows. I used to run away from ebbs and flows, wanting them to be over as soon as possible. I remember once going through a very difficult time. This was in my early twenties when I was struggling with depression. I was empty, having lost joy in life, and I couldn't sleep. It was a very hard time for me. It took time for me to get to a point where I accepted 100 percent that I was not well and became willing to fight to feel better again. I wanted to laugh again and be happy. I remembered back to my teenage years, recalling a sentence that I kept writing in my journal and that I carried deep inside. I had lost touch with this sentence, and I wanted to reconnect with it: "I feel so much love within me, which is ready to be shared."

The moment I started to accept that I was not well, the moment when I was finally ready to embrace the ebbs in my life, was the biggest game-changer of my life. Instead of blocking myself, I let the energy flow. I felt the emotions in my body. The healing was allowed to enter. I opened the door for healing. Having left the door open, I was ready for a miracle. I was ready to receive wonderful things, and I did. I worked on myself for months and began to feel greater joy and gratitude for myself and life that I had never allowed myself to feel before. I was ready for life and for all that it had to offer me. And life had something wonderful to offer. The love I had inside me and was ready to share found me. I met my husband during that time. I found love and it found me.

Allow yourself to embrace the ebbs in your life. Allow yourself to feel and accept the bad moments in your life. Do not block yourself. Be willing to learn from the bad moments in your life. Be willing to go through the bad moments in your life and, by accepting them, open the door to the most wonderful moments you will ever experience.

Remember, after an ebb tide comes a flood tide. Without a low tide, there would be no high tide. Go with the flow of life. Don't run away. Let yourself glide, and always keep your doors open.

Honor Your Body

Honoring my body helped me very much to be at peace with myself. Every day I connect with my body and honor it. In so doing, I take the moment to feel gratitude for my body and all it does. By doing this every day, I started to feel very much at peace with myself. I connected on a new level with my body. I started to see myself in a new light; I talked differently to myself; I became gentler with myself. I simply started to love myself in a much deeper way than I ever had before.

I would like to share some simple and effective tools with you today so that you can start to connect with your body on a deeper level too. These tools will help you practice honoring your body and finding gratitude for it. It does not take long. You will see that the more you follow these easy steps and incorporate them into your daily life, the more you will feel at peace with yourself. You will become gentler with yourself and will find love for yourself.

1. Find Gratitude for Your Body

Honor Your Body

We demand so much from our bodies every day. Our days are filled with tasks that need to be done, and our bodies run at full speed in the effort to complete these tasks. Our bodies do their best every day to keep us functioning.

When was the last time you said thank you to your body?

We take for granted that we can walk, that we breathe, that our food is digested. But the body works hard to do these things.

Take a moment each day to connect with your body and find gratitude for it. Give it a moment of attention. Believe me, it will thank you. Your body will keep the energy from the gratitude that you give it each day. The more it gets, the more it will have to give back to you.

Set a timer or practice a moment of gratitude for your body first thing in the morning. You will see that this small moment can make a big difference in your daily life.

2. Nourish Your Body with the Right Food

As mentioned in chapter 3 and also earlier in this chapter, you can do a lot with your food choices. By choosing food that supports your body and your digestion and provides energy, not taking it away, you provide your body with everything it needs to function optimally. It is supplied with important nutrients, including vitamins and minerals, that it needs to go through the day full of energy and health. Your mood will be positively influenced, along with your whole well-being, when you choose nutritious foods.

3. Focus on the Rhythm of Your Body

It is perfectly normal to have days when you have less energy and motivation than others. These days are important. Honor them. Embrace these days and take it slow. Your body needs this time. As mentioned, when discussing the ebbs and flows of life earlier in this chapter, it is important that you embrace these days and allow yourself to have them. Don't run away these days. The body has its own rhythm. Embrace that rhythm. Allow yourself quieter moments or quieter days.

It is all about balance. Find your balance. Live in alignment and with the rhythm of your body, not against it.

4. Feel Your Emotions

As important as it is to listen to your body and live in its rhythm, it is equally important to feel your emotions. Don't run away from your emotions. Allow yourself to feel them. Let them come up so they can be processed instead of just sitting in your body. It's important to feel the emotions in your body. Give yourself permission to be sad or to be angry. However, it is important that you not remain in your head. In your head, you find only the stories that your ego tells you about your situation. Becoming healthy is about allowing yourself to feel. Feel where in your body the sadness, the anger, or whatever other emotion presents itself. I once read that ninety second is enough to feel the emotion. Take those ninety seconds and feel the emotion so that it can dissolve and leave your body.

All it takes is being in the here and now. Be present, feel your emotions, and connect to your body.

5. Always Be Gentle with Yourself

This mantra has become my best friend over the years. I spent many years demanding a lot from my body. I was an absolute perfectionist, never completely satisfied with what I was doing, how I was doing it, or what my body was like. By growing in self-love, I found that my attitude toward myself changed. The more I began to love my body and listen to it, the more my energy changed. I gradually put away that "push" energy, the energy driving me to always do more, never being satisfied. I made room for a warm, nurturing, and soft energy. Of course, still have moments today when that push energy comes back. I am human, so it is perfectly normal to fall back into my old patterns. The key is to recognize these patterns early. This is done by being present. By being present, and being in the moment, I am able to recognize these patterns. I then remember my mantra: "Be gentle with yourself."

This mantra brings me back to the now and helps me shift my energy. It helps me to realign my perspective.

Allow yourself to be gentle with yourself too. Less is more. You've probably heard this phrase too. Give yourself permission to believe that less is more. Believe that you can reach your goal much more easily and simply with less. Do not block yourself by pushing and forcing something; instead, let your energy flow. Listen to your body, to its pace and energy, and let it guide you.

Love yourself as you are. Accept yourself as you are. Remember, you are exactly where you need to be. You are unique. You are perfect just as you are. Enjoy the perfectly imperfect. None of us is really perfect. It may seem by the outward appearance that some people are perfect, but we don't know what goes on behind closed doors. Maybe the person you see as perfect admires you as much as you admire them.

Embrace yourself. Love yourself the way you want to be loved by others. You have the opportunity to give yourself unconditional love. You are here for a reason. Like all of us, you have a light inside you that is ready to shine. Don't hide from anything. Be brave and spread your light and your love. Follow your true purpose. Always listen to your heart and your intuition. They are your guides. They are here to show you the way you are meant to go. All you have to do is to be and live in the present moment, love yourself, listen to yourself, and take care of yourself.

Everything will be okay in the end. If it is not, then it is not the end.

I have lived by this mantra for as long as I can remember, and I share it with my children all the time. Even as a little girl, I knew that everything would be okay. Too many times I was trapped in my head. I am very emotional and tend to get lost in my emotions, a typical Cancer trait. This mantra has always brought me back to reality. It has been with me since I can remember, and it has proven to be true again and again.

May this mantra also accompany you. May it be your new daily companion, leading you out of dark moments and back into the light. Never lose faith in the good. You are here to experience good and to do good. You are here to show your light. Be brave, go your own way, and shine your light. Never forget: Everything will be okay in the end. If not, then it is not the end.

Trust that you are guided. Trust that you are so much more than you think you are. You are unique. There is only one person on this earth with your fingerprints. There is only one you. Never forget how unique you are. Embrace your uniqueness. Never let anyone or anything dim your inner light. Keep your light lit in dark moments as well as in bright moments. Never forget that everything is here for a reason. Everything happens for a reason, and you are supposed to learn from everything that happens, so you can grow and become the best version of yourself. Everything happening to you is happening for a purpose. Trust the bigger picture. Stay open to magic, and it will find you.

Trust your guidance and trust life. Be open to life and be open to living your best life ever.

6

Nourish Yourself with Self-Love, Food, and Spirituality—Final Word

The title of my book is also my intention for the book. Each and every one of us is unique. That is our power and, at the same time, our gift. There is no one in the world who has the same fingerprint as you. Always be aware of your uniqueness. You alone know what is best for you. When you connect with your body and your intuition, learning to speak the language of your body and your intuition, you will always know what is best for you.

Nourish yourself with self-love, food, and spirituality. You have only one body, and it is your temple, your tool to go your way while you're here on earth. It accompanies you and is always there for you. Nourish it with the best possible energy. Give your body attention and love and nourish it with foods that help it to function optimally.

If you give a car the wrong gasoline, it won't run properly. The same is true for your body. Give it the right gasoline; be good to it. And always remember, each of us is unique and therefore needs the best nourishment when it comes to self-care, self-love, food, and spirituality. What is right for you may not be right for your loved ones.

Stay present, go inward, and connect with yourself on a daily basis. What can you do every day to support yourself and your body and be your best self? You deserve to feel good, be happy, and shine every day.

Keep telling yourself that you love yourself. Never forget that where you are is exactly where you need to be. Trust your own path. Have faith in the bigger picture. Never forget: Everything will be okay in the end. If it is not, then it is not the end.

You are doing your best, whatever that looks like for you. You are writing your book here on earth, and each chapter is exactly the way it is meant to be.

Never stop shining your light. Never stop being in your power. Never stop being you.

You are unique.

You are here for a reason.

There is no one else on this planet like you.

You are love.

You are beautiful.

7

Nourishing Recipes

Food is a very big part of my life. Food is energy to the body. As *Nourish Yourself* is about energy, the body, and the connection between the two, I have chosen to share my favorite recipes on these pages. The recipes found here are my favorites. I eat these foods all the time. They nourish my body and soul with beautiful energy, and I hope they will do the same for you.

As mentioned earlier, I am all about getting back to basics and doing simple things when it comes to food. An apple or an avocado does not need to be advertised for you to know that it is good for you. Food from nature, pure and full of the best nutrients, is what your body needs.

My recipes are all easy to make. They require little time and few ingredients. If there is an ingredient you don't have or don't like, simply replace it. Change up the recipe if you feel like it.

It is important that you are satisfied with your food and that it nourishes your body. To me, a meal has to make me happy. This is my intention for being in the kitchen and creating recipes. I want everyone making my recipes to feel happy, satisfied, and nourished.

Smoothies and Juices

Debora's Basic Hydrating Green Juice

This is one of my favorite juices. I drink it first thing in the morning. It is hydrating and gives me energy for the day.

1 serving

Ingredients
1 green apple
5 stalks celery
1 cucumber
small piece gingerroot

Preparation
Wash all ingredients. Put them through the juicer. Pour into a glass.

Green Goddess Smoothie

This is my absolute favorite green smoothie. Especially during the colder months, I love to start my day with a green smoothie, which nourishes my whole body and gives it lots of energy.

2–3 servings

Ingredients
2–3 large handfuls of lamb's lettuce or spinach
4 stalks celery
1/3 cucumber
juice of 1/2 lemon
400–500 milliliters of water
1 tablespoon spirulina (optional)
1 banana
1/2 apple
1/4 bunch parsley

Preparation
Blend lettuce in a powerful blender. Cut celery and cucumber into small pieces. Blend. Add lemon juice, water, and spirulina and blend well. Cut apple and banana into small pieces, add the fruits to your smoothie mixture, and blend well. Pour into 3 glasses if serving immediately. Will keep in a sealed container in the refrigerator for 1–2 days.

Unrepentant Nourishing and Sweet Chocolate Smoothie

A sweet warming hug to start your day

This smoothie is one of my favorites when I want something sweet but still want to nourish my body. I normally drink it in the afternoon as it keeps me satisfied. However, it is perfect any time of the day, especially for those who love a sweet but still healthy and nourishing drink.

1 serving

Ingredients
180 milliliters of oat milk or almond milk
1 banana
1 Medjool date
1 tablespoon almond butter or nut butter of choice
1 tablespoon sugar-free cacao powder

Preparation
Blend all ingredients listed in a powerful blender. Pour directly into a smoothie glass and enjoy.

Nourishing Breakfast Bowls

Debora's Signature Wellness Fruit Bowl

A nourishing fruity treat for your body and soul

I love to eat a fruit bowl in the morning. I always go for seasonal fruits. My signature bowl is full of healthy nutrients, including vitamins, minerals, and fiber. It provides my body with lots of energy to start the day. Also, fruit contains a lot of water, which is very hydrating for the body—especially important in the morning.

1 serving

Ingredients
1 apple
1/2–1 banana
2–3 handfuls of berries (raspberries, strawberries, blueberries)
80 milliliters of coconut water
2 heaping tablespoons of natural coconut yogurt (about 60 grams)
1 tablespoon cacao nibs
cinnamon to taste

Preparation
Chop the apple and banana and put them in a cereal bowl. Add berries. Sprinkle coconut water over the fruits. Top with coconut yogurt and cacao nibs. Sprinkle with cinnamon.

Porridges and Overnight Oats

Back-to-Basics Almond Porridge

This is my favorite porridge, easy to make and delicious. It takes just a few minutes to prepare, and it is satisfying and nourishing.

1 serving

Ingredients
40–50 grams fine rolled oats
2 cups water or plant milk of choice
1/2 tablespoon chia seeds
cinnamon to taste
2–3 tablespoons coconut yogurt
1 tablespoon almond paste
One handful chopped almonds

Preparation
In a saucepan, heat oatmeal with water or plant milk and chia seeds. Simmer over low heat. Stir frequently. Add cinnamon. As soon as the liquid is absorbed, stir in the yogurt and almond paste. Pour into a bowl. Garnish with chopped almonds.

Tip: Roast the almonds if you prefer before you put them on your porridge.

Creamy Overnight Oats

A creamy way to start your day

For anyone who loves creamy oats or has no time to make breakfast, these overnight oats are very easy to make, along with being delicious and satisfying.

2 servings

Ingredients
80–100 grams rolled oats
1 tablespoon chia seeds
2 tablespoons almond paste
1 teaspoon cinnamon
1 banana, mashed
4 tablespoons coconut yogurt
200 milliliters almond milk or oat milk
toppings of your choice

Preparation
Place oats and chia seeds in a bowl. Add almond paste and cinnamon. Stir well. Mash banana with a fork. Add to oatmeal mixture. Add coconut yogurt and plant milk. Stir again well. Cover the bowl and it put in the refrigerator for a few hours or overnight. Serve with toppings of your choice.

Basic Chocolate Porridge

This is for all the chocolate fans. I love this porridge. Whenever I feel like eating more than just a basic porridge, I go for this creamy chocolate version. It is very easy to make and nourishing to the soul.

2 servings

Ingredients
80 grams rolled oats
2 tablespoons chia seeds
2 deciliters oat milk or almond milk
2 deciliters water
1 teaspoon cinnamon
1–2 tablespoons cacao powder
1–2 tablespoons maple syrup (optional)

Preparation
In a saucepan, heat oats, chia seeds, oat milk or almond milk, water, and cinnamon until liquid is absorbed, stirring well. Add cacao powder and maple syrup and stir again. Heat for 2 minutes. Serve in bowls with toppings of your choice.

Tip: For creamier porridge, fold in some coconut yogurt.

Debora's Wellness Sugar-Free Granolas

I love granolas. I eat homemade granolas all the time. I love it on top of my porridge with coconut yogurt or as a topping for my deserts. I truly can't live without granola.

Simple Cinnamon Cashew Granola

If you are a granola lover too, you will love this. Crunchy and sugar-free, it still has a sweet taste because of the cinnamon and cashews.

Ingredients

60 grams of rolled oats
15 grams of quinoa pops
1 teaspoon cinnamon
30 grams cashew nuts, chopped
1/2 banana, mashed
1 heaping tablespoon cashew butter

Preparation

In a bowl, combine rolled oats, quinoa pops, and cinnamon. Add cashews to the cereal bowl and combine. In a small bowl, mash the banana with a fork and mix it with the cashew butter. Then put it over your cereals and mix everything well together. Then place the mixture on a baking tray lined with parchment paper. Bake in a convection oven at 150 degrees for 15 minutes.

Tip: For sweeter granola, add some coconut syrup or maple syrup to the banana nut mixture.

Debora's Wellness Basic Granola

Ninety percent of the time when I eat granola, this is the recipe I use. I have tried many different ones, but I always come back to this one. It is sugar-free and crunchy, and the banana and almond make it sweet.

Ingredients
100 grams rolled oats
30 grams quinoa pops
1 teaspoon cinnamon
30 grams coconut chips
1 banana, mashed
2 tablespoons almond paste
60 grams almonds, chopped

Preparation
In a medium bowl, stir together oats, quinoa pops, almonds, cinnamon, and coconut chips. Mash the banana and combine with almond paste, then add to the dry mixture. Stir everything well. Put the mixture on a baking tray lined with parchment paper. Bake at 150 degrees for 15–20 minutes.

Tip: For sweeter granola, add some coconut syrup or maple syrup to the banana nut mixture.

Savory Breakfast or Snack Ideas

*A Nourishing Piece of Heaven
for Your Body and Soul*

Debora's Wellness Beauty Bread

*Beauty starts on the inside. Shine
from the inside out*

I am obsessed with this bread, which I eat several times a week as a side dish to the salad I make for lunch or as a snack. The cucumber hydrates the skin; the nutrient-dense sprouts fill the body with youthful energy, and the cream cheese or avocado provides healthy fat to benefit the skin and the hormones.

Ingredients
2 slices sourdough or pumpernickel bread
2 tablespoons vegan cashew cream cheese or avocado
1 handful sprouts of your choice
a few slices of cucumber
half a lemon or lime
optional: a little bit of sea salt

Preparation
If you use avocado you can take a fork and mash the avocado before you put it on your toast. Then put your bread into a toaster and as soon as it is ready, put your mashed avocado or vegan cream cheese on the toast and top it with the cucumber slices and sprouts of your choice. Squeeze your lemon or lime over the toast and enjoy.

Perfect Snack to Go—Simple Avocado Tomato Sandwich

A little treat on the way is never a bad thing

This recipe is very easy to make and tastes very good. Whenever you have limited time in the morning, it is the perfect breakfast go-to. I am all about simple foods that keep me full and satisfied and also nourish my body with amazing nutrients.

Ingredients
1/2 avocado
seasoning of choice
lemon juice to taste
2 slices of sourdough bread
1 tomato
lettuce leaves or basil leaves (optional)

Preparation
Mash the avocado with a fork in a bowl. Season to taste and add lemon juice to it. Spread mixture on slices of bread. Slice tomato and place on bread slices. Add lettuce or basil if you like.

Salads

Simple Tomato Avocado Salad with Chickpeas

Simply delicious

I am very big on salads. Normally, I include a large portion of leafy greens. However, this combination of tomato and chickpeas is one of my favorites too. I enjoy having it now and then in place of a salad with leafy greens.

2 servings

Ingredients
Salad
1 jar of cooked chickpeas (200 grams)
2 handfuls of cherry tomatoes or 2 large tomatoes
1 avocado
parsley for garnish

Dressing
2 tablespoons olive oil
2 tablespoons apple cider vinegar
1 tablespoon dry salad herbs
pepper to taste
herbed salt to taste
2 tablespoons water

Preparation
For the Salad
Dice tomatoes and avocado and put them in a bowl. Add the chickpeas and combine everything together.

For the Dressing

In a small bowl, combine oil, vinegar, herbed salt, pepper, and water. Pour it over the salad and mix it all well together. Garnish with parsley.

Sweet Peanut Butter Zoodle Salad

A little bit of Asia in your home

Given that my husband is of Asian ethnicity, we often eat Asian food. This one is my own creation. Whenever I feel like having Asian food, I make this salad. My husband and I are truly obsessed with it.

2 servings

Ingredients
1 cucumber, washed
2–3 large carrots, washed and peeled
dry salad herbs
2 tablespoons balsamic vinegar
2 tablespoons olive oil
1 tablespoon maple syrup (optional)
2 tablespoons peanut butter
2 tablespoons water
One handful of peanuts, chopped
cilantro, chopped

Preparation
With a spiral cutter, make noodles of the carrots and cucumbers. Place it in a bowl. In a food processor, small shaker, or blender, blend herbs, peanut butter, balsamic vinegar, and olive oil. Add maple syrup, peanut butter, and water to it and blend again until it gets creamy. Pour sauce over noodles. Fold in peanuts and cilantro. Serve on plates.

Debora's Back-to-Basics Wellness Green Superfood Salad

Simply beauty on a plate

This is the way I love to have my salad, with a mix of leafy greens and toppings.

2 servings

Ingredients
Salad
3 or 4 handfuls of leafy greens of choice
2 tablespoons sunflower seeds
2 tablespoons hemp seeds
chopped parsley
2–4 radishes, chopped
A small handful of sprouts of your choice

Dressing
2 tablespoons virgin olive oil
2 tablespoons apple cider vinegar
dry salad herbs of your choice
2 tablespoons of water

Preparation
Place your greens on your plates. In a small bowl, combine olive oil, apple cider vinegar, herbs, and water. Pour it over your greens. Top with sunflower seeds, hemp seeds, parsley, radishes, and sprouts. Serve and enjoy.

Lunch / Dinner

These are my favorite recipes that I cook for myself and my family. They are made within no time and they support your body with beautiful energy.

Chickpea Turmeric Curry

A warm hug for your whole body

This curry is one of my favorites for the colder months. It truly warms my soul, and the turmeric is very beneficial to the digestive system.

3–4 servings

Ingredients
2 cups basmati, jasmine, or brown rice
5 deciliters coconut milk
1 teaspoon turmeric powder
2 teaspoons curry powder
1 bunch broccoli, chopped
2–3 carrots, chopped
200 grams cooked chickpeas
50 grams of bean sprouts (optional)

Preparation
Cook your rice according to instructions. Meanwhile, stir coconut milk and spices in a pan. Heat to a simmer. Add broccoli and carrots. Simmer until vegetables are firm to the bite (about 10-15 Minutes). Add the chickpeas for the last 2-3 Minutes and let it cook on low heat.

Serve on plates and top it with bean sprouts if you like.

Lettuce Wraps with Lentils and Vegetables

This recipe has it all: greens, lots of healthy protein, and healthy carbs from the lentils. It supports digestion thanks to the celery, and the coconut oil provides healthy fat needed by the hormones and the whole body.

2 servings

Ingredients

4 stalks celery
1 large carrot
1 zucchini
1/2 onion
1 tablespoon coconut oil
120 grams lentils
500 milliliters of vegetable broth, divided
8–10 large lettuce leaves
3–4 tablespoons vegan cream cheese
black pepper to taste (optional)
sea salt to taste (optional)

Preparation

Chop celery, carrot, and zucchini. Set aside. In a pan, sauté onion with coconut oil until translucent. Add chopped vegetables. Sauté for 4–5 minutes. Add the lentils and deglaze with 300 milliliters of the vegetable broth. Simmer over low heat for thirty minutes, until lentils are tender. Add remainder of vegetable broth if liquid evaporates.

Wash lettuce leaves and put them on a large plate. Spread with vegan cream cheese. Then add lentil mixture to it and enjoy.

Debora's Wellness Quinoa Bowl

I love this dish and eat it frequently. You can choose any vegetables you like. I normally use whatever greens I have in my fridge. Basically just mix quinoa, veggies, lemon, almond or nut butter, and olive oil, and season to taste. It is simple and good and truly gives your body all it needs.

2 servings

Ingredients

2 cups quinoa
100 grams of frozen peas
1 bunch broccoli, chopped
1 tablespoon olive oil
1 tablespoon almond paste
black pepper to taste
sea salt to taste
2 tablespoons chopped almonds
parsley for garnish
a handful of arugula for garnish
the juice of half a lemon

Preparation

Cook quinoa according to instructions. Wash the broccoli and cut it. Then add the broccoli with some water (just as much that the broccoli is almost covered with water) in a pan and cook it for 5-7 minutes. For the last two minutes add the peas. In a bowl, combine olive oil, almond paste, pepper, and sea salt. Combine the quinoa with the vegetables. Fold in almond paste mixture. Garnish with almonds, parsley, and arugula. Sprinkle with the lemon juice.

Lentil Bolognese

I love to cook this on the weekends. It is very good and may be served with any kind of pasta. My family and I eat a lot of pasta. Topped with this lentil Bolognese, it is a very warming, nourishing meat-free meal.

3–4 servings

Ingredients
1/2 onion, chopped
coconut oil
2 carrots, chopped
4 stalks of celery, chopped
2 cans of diced organic tomatoes (about 400 grams for one can)
200 grams lentils
about 400 milliliters of vegetable broth, divided
some dry Italian herbs for the spice
sea salt and pepper to taste

Preparation
In a pan, sauté onion in coconut oil until translucent. Wash the carrots and the celery and cut them into small pieces. Then add carrots and celery to the pan. Sauté for about 3-5 minutes. Add tomatoes, lentils, and 250–300 milliliters of vegetable broth. Add herbs, salt, and pepper to taste. Simmer over low heat, stirring frequently, until lentils are soft, about half an hour. Add the remaining vegetable broth if the liquid evaporates.

Healthy Sweets

If you are like me, you let no day go by without eating a healthy treat. I love chocolate. Here I am sharing some of my absolute go-to treats. They are refined-sugar-free and are still very satisfying and sweet.

Simple Vegan No-Bake Hazelnut Brownies

Nuts meet chocolate—heaven

What can I say, I love hazelnuts and chocolate. To me, this is the perfect combination and simply a piece of heaven.

12 pieces

Ingredients
Brownies
15 soft Medjool dates
200 grams hazelnuts
4 tablespoons cacao
Pinch of sea salt

Glaze
4 tablespoons cacao powder
3–4 tablespoons maple syrup
4 tablespoons almond milk or nut milk of your choice
40 grams hazelnut paste

Preparation

For the Brownies

Mix dates, hazelnuts, salt, and raw cacao powder in a food processor. Press it into a baking dish (I use one of 24 x 15 cm) and set it aside.

For the Glaze

Combine cacao powder, maple syrup, nut milk, and hazelnut paste. Then spread it on the brownie mixture.

Put your baking dish in the refrigerator for 1–2 hours. Remove it from the refrigerator and cut brownies into squares.

Sinful Sweet Hot Chocolate without Sugar

Everyone who knows me personally or follows me on Instagram knows I can't live without my hot chocolate. Here is one of the ways I prepare it. To me, drinking hot chocolate is the perfect way to practice a moment of self-care on a busy day.

2 servings

Ingredients
200 milliliters water
250 milliliters of oat milk or almond milk
2 1/2 tablespoons cacao powder
3 tablespoons almond paste
4 Medjool dates
1/2 teaspoon cinnamon

Preparation
Put the dates, cinnamon, cacao powder, milk, water, and nut paste all in a blender and blend until creamy. Put it then into a small pan and heat it up until your chocolate gets warm. Let it simmer for 5–10 minutes.

Pour it then into 2 cups. Serve and enjoy.

Tip: This recipe is very tasty when cooled. Place in a sealed container and store in the refrigerator for up to two days. The chocolate becomes even creamier.

Banana Crumble with Chocolate Sauce

The perfect combination of crunchy and sweet

Are you also a big fan of crumbles? If so, then this one is a must. I love it. It has the perfect combination of crunchiness and sweetness.

2 servings

Ingredients
2 bananas
2–3 Medjool dates, chopped
1 tablespoon coconut syrup or maple syrup (optional)

Crumble
15 grams rolled oats
25 grams flour of choice (I use buckwheat flour or almond flour)
15 grams of chopped almonds or chopped nuts of choice
1/2 teaspoon cinnamon
1/2 teaspoon vanilla
2 tablespoons coconut oil
1 tablespoon coconut syrup or maple syrup (optional)

Sauce
1.5 tablespoons cacao powder
1 tablespoon maple syrup
6 tablespoons plant-based milk of choice

Preparation
Slice bananas and put them in a baking dish (I use one which is 19 x 14 cm). Cut your dates into pieces and put them over the bananas. Add the syrup and mix it all together.

For the Crumble

In a bowl, combine flour and oats, then add nuts, cinnamon, and vanilla. Stir everything. In a small pan, heat coconut oil over low heat until melted. Allow to cool and mix it with the syrup. Put the syrup over the dry ingredients and stir everything until large crumbs form. Spread crumble on the banana mixture.

Bake at 150 degrees for 10–12 minutes.

For the Sauce

Combine raw persimmon powder, maple syrup, and coconut water. Drizzle over the crumble.

Tip: Substitute vegan yogurt or ice cream for chocolate sauce.

Easy Cookies with just 5 ingredients
(Vegan and Gluten-Free)

A cookie and a glass of milk? I'm there.

These cookies are one of my favorites. They are gluten-free and sugar-free and are easy to prepare with little time or effort. Does it get any better than this?

14 pieces

Ingredients
6 Medjool dates
140 grams almonds
1 tablespoon chia seeds
60 milliliters of nut milk of your choice
60 grams of chopped chocolate of your choice (I choose vegan chocolate with 85 percent or more cacao, sweetened with coconut nectar)

Preparation
If necessary, soak the dates in water to soften. Add dates and almonds to a food processor. Grind everything. Add chia seeds and nut milk. Blend it and fold in the chopped chocolate.

Using a large spoon, drop by the spoonful onto a baking tray lined with parchment paper. Bake at 180 degrees celsius for 10–12 minutes.

Stuffed Dates

This is my go-to snack when I need something truly filling and don't have much time. I always have dates, cacao nibs, and almond butter at home. These stuffed dates are very good and keep you full and satisfied for hours. This truly is back to basics to me.

4 pieces

Ingredients
4 Medjool dates
2 tablespoons almond paste
2 tablespoons cacao nibs

Preparation
Cut the dates with a knife. Divide the almond paste into four even portions. Fill each date with a portion of almond paste. Top each date with cacao nibs.

Debora's Wellness Vegan Gluten-Free and Sugar-Free Banana Bread

This last recipe is another signature recipe. I created this banana bread once out of just what I had at home. It turned out to be delicious, so I decided to name it "Debora's Wellness"—and I had to share it here. It is something I can eat anytime—for breakfast, for snack, or as a side dish as part of a bigger meal.

Ingredients

4 ripe bananas, mashed with a fork

100 milliliters of coconut oil
1 teaspoon cinnamon
1/2 teaspoon vanilla powder
60 milliliters oat milk or plant milk of choice
50 grams of quinoa flour or buckwheat flour
1 teaspoon baking powder
220 grams gluten-free rolled oats (alternatively, normal rolled oats), ground to flour consistency
100 grams of almond flour

Preparation

Melt the coconut oil in a pan and let it cool down. Then add the banana, cinnamon, and vanilla powder. Blend or whisk everything together. Add nut milk and stir. In a small bowl, combine the flour (almond and buckwheat or quinoa), your oat flour, and baking powder. Next, add the banana mixture to the flour mixture. Stir until combined.

Grease a cake pan. Pour in the batter. Bake in a convection oven at 180 degrees C for 35–40 minutes.

Acknowledgments

I was able to write *Nourish Yourself* thanks to my family and some of my greatest teachers in life. I dedicate this work to all of you.

My kids: Being my greatest teachers, you always motivate me to be the best version of myself. The love you give me every day is the greatest thing I know. The curiosity and inspiration that I see in your eyes every day not only motivates me to always have motivation and inspiration but also causes me to want to discover the world and see it openly and be full of curiosity.

My husband: For fourteen years, you have been my companion. You have accepted me as I am every day and every second. I have great respect for you and am very grateful to have someone like you by my side. I am grateful that you always make me feel that I and our children are the most important things to you. I am thankful for the wonderful words you have for me after fourteen years and the love you give me. I am thankful that you always support me 100 percent in everything. Thank you for your love!

Kimberly Snyder: You are a true inspiration. I am very thankful that I found your books. When I decided to change my diet, I found my way to your books. I still enjoy drinking the GGS today. Not only did you bring the green smoothie into my life, but also you taught me so much about nutrition. Your books helped me get the ball rolling, and I subsequently became more and more involved with nutrition and especially digestion. Thanks to you, I am now an integrative nutrition health coach. Your work is wonderful, and your heart and energy impel people to find their light and share it with the world.

Gabby Bernstein: I am so incredibly grateful that I found your book *The Universe Has Your Back* a few years ago. More likely, it found me. Since then, not a day has gone by that I haven't meditated. Your work is wonderful. You are a gift to this world. Thank you for showing me the way to spirituality. Thank you for being. Thank you for all you do for so many people. Thank you for finding me and inspiring me again and again.

Bondi Guru: I am beyond grateful that I found you on social media in 2020. Your work helped me to strengthen my intuition and to learn to know and love myself on a much deeper level. Please continue with your daily intuitive horoscopes. They are my go-to every day.

Mum: Thank you for encouraging me to write when I was a little girl. I'll never forget the moment you printed out my essay and auditioned it. That made me feel special. It gave me courage, inspiration, love, and joy.

My kindergarten teacher: I will never forget the picture book of the little dormouse hoping to meet Santa Claus. This picture book has been my absolute favorite book since kindergarten. It was through this book that I found my love for books.

Vanessa: I am beyond thankful that I met you. I am very thankful for your help and for the fact that you always have an open ear for me. No matter how much is going on in your life, you are always there for me. This means the world to me.

Daniela: I am very happy and thankful that after all these years we found each other again. To me, our friendship does not need many words. We are very much energetically connected, and that is something I love. Thank you for always having an open ear, and thank you very much for always asking how I am doing.

To all my readers: Thank you for reading my blog posts. Thank you for your wonderful feedback. It warms my heart and gives me love, motivation, and the confidence to be on the right path and do something good.

Universe: Dear universe, thank you for having my back. Thank you for guiding me, showing me the way to go, and supporting me no matter what. Thank you for writing, speaking, moving, acting, and talking through me. Thank you for helping me to be of service and showing me how.

Hay House: I am beyond thankful that through Hay House I found Balboa Press. Thank you so much for helping me bring this book to light and accessible for everyone who wants to read it. Thank you for your help and support along my journey to write this book.

Are you curious to find out more about my journey and Deboras Wellness?

Find more on my website: https://deboraswellness.ch/
or on my Instagram @deboraswellness

Thank you from my heart for letting me be a part of your journey and for reading NOURISH YOURSELF! Lots of love from me to you.

About the Author

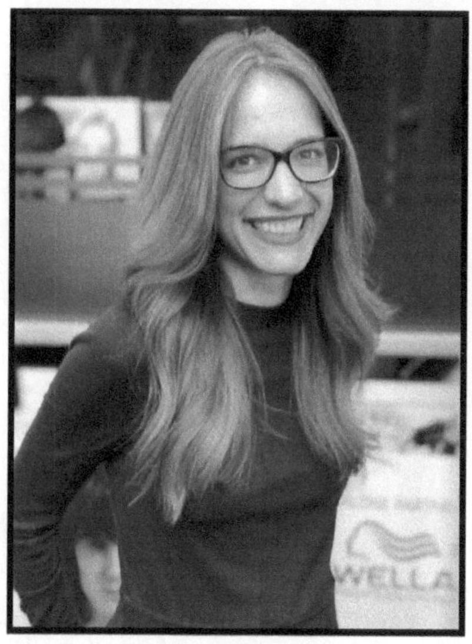

Debora Accola is a integrative nutrition health coach, yoga and pilates teacher. Her work is all about connection to your inner power, learn to listen to your intuition and your body and find love for yourself. Find out more online about Debora and her work: https://deboraswellness.ch/